The Family Experience of Dementia

of related interest

Young Onset Dementia
A Guide to Recognition, Diagnosis, and Supporting Individuals with Dementia and Their Families
Hilda Hayo, Alison Ward, and Jacqueline Parkes
Foreword by Wendy Mitchell
ISBN 978 1 78592 117 9
eISBN 978 1 78450 383 3

Timely Psychosocial Interventions in Dementia Care
Evidence-Based Practice
Edited by Jill Manthorpe and Esme Moniz-Cook
Foreword by Helen Rochford-Brennan, Chairperson of the European Working Group of People with Dementia
ISBN 978 1 78775 302 0
eISBN 978 1 78775 303 7

Promoting Resilience in Dementia Care
A Person-Centred Framework for Assessment and Support Planning
Julie Christie
Forewords by Wendy Mitchell and Mary Marshall
ISBN 978 1 78592 600 6
eISBN 978 1 78592 601 3

Understanding Behaviour in Dementia that Challenges
A Guide to Assessment and Treatment
Ian Andrew James
ISBN 978 1 84905 108 8
eISBN 978 0 85700 296 9

Dementia – Support for Family and Friends, Second Edition
Dave Pulsford and Rachel Thompson
ISBN 978 1 78592 437 8
eISBN 978 1 78450 811 1

The Family Experience of Dementia

A Reflective Workbook for Professionals

JACK MORRIS and GARY MORRIS

Foreword by Kate Swaffer

Jessica Kingsley Publishers
London and Philadelphia

First published in Great Britain in 2021 by Jessica Kingsley Publishers
An Hachette Company

1

Front cover image source: frimages/iStock®.

A CIP catalogue record for this title is available from the British Library and the Library of Congress

ISBN 978 1 78592 574 0
eISBN 978 1 78450 983 5

Printed and bound in Great Britain by Clays Ltd

Jessica Kingsley Publishers' policy is to use papers that are natural, renewable and recyclable products and made from wood grown in sustainable forests. The logging and manufacturing processes are expected to conform to the environmental regulations of the country of origin.

Jessica Kingsley Publishers
Carmelite House
50 Victoria Embankment
London EC4Y 0DZ

www.jkp.com

(Jack)

To: Pamela

With much love

(Gary)

To: Emily, Daisy and Caitlin

Lottie, William, Sam,

With much love

&

Manfred Maier

Michael Blackwell

Stanislav Lodowski

Fondly remembered

Contents

Foreword

It was with some trepidation I read this book, in particular because it says I have inspired the authors. Although this is gratifying, it definitely adds some pressure to my past work and writings, and also to my theories on what it is really like living with a diagnosis of dementia.

This book offers a series of narratives from people who themselves are diagnosed with dementia, and from many others including care partners and families of people living with dementia. It challenges some of the negative narrative and thinking about us and provides me with hope.

The only people who can truly describe what it is like living with dementia are those of us who are diagnosed with it. Families, care partners, children and others who support and live alongside us have their own unique but separate journeys. This book explores the multi-varied experiences involved in living with and alongside dementia. It provides readers with positive messages and learnings connected with these experiences.

As I was quoted saying in 2012, 'There is a gross underestimation of the capacities of all people with dementia', and I believe this book will help everyone to understand this to be true. As a workbook for professionals, this is an essential outcome.

'Living beyond dementia', a term I have been using for almost a decade, quickly describes that people diagnosed with dementia do not simply need to go home and prepare to die. With disability support, and a major change in attitudes towards and about us, we can live meaningful and productive lives. It does not mean we were misdiagnosed, nor does it mean dementia is not a terminal illness. It does however mean we are still people, and we are very much still here and if we ignore the Prescribed Disengagement®, which is all we are offered at the time of diagnosis and after, we can live a more positive life than once thought. We may be changing, but we are just changing in ways that people without dementia are not.

Hence, although when I was first diagnosed with dementia I wrote about my disappearing world, I did not disappear; that world has gone due to the loss of identity due primarily to losing my job, and to the pervasive stigma and discrimination, but my life is still full of meaning and achievements.

This workbook will help you all see the person, not the dementia, and will inspire you to change your attitude, your practice, and most of all, I hope it will inspire you to support people with dementia to live positively with their diagnosis, for as long as possible, rather than only support them to go home and wait to die from it.

Kate Swaffer, MSc, BPsych, BA, retired nurse,
author, poet, disability activist and Humanitarian Chair,
CEO and Co-Founder of Dementia Alliance International
Website and blog: https://kateswaffer.com/daily-blog

Acknowledgements

The authors would like to extend their thanks to a number of people who have provided invaluable assistance to the development and production of this work.

Jessica Kingsley Publishers: Elen Griffiths, Sarah Hamlin, Karina Maduro and Emma Scriver for your support and guidance at all stages of this project as well as your understanding and rapid response when further help (and time) was needed.

Practitioners: Nicky Needham, Richard Clibbens and Alex Hart for your enthusiasm, vibrant discussions and wonderful contributions to the associated dementia learning module at the University of Leeds.

Students: nursing students at the University of Leeds for your active engagement with this developing work and thoughtful discussions. This has greatly aided the direction we have subsequently taken in developing core themes.

Daisy Morris and Tim Morris: for your fabulous illustrations xx

Copyright Acknowledgements

Ten early symptoms of dementia list on p.36 is reproduced with kind permission of Alzheimer's Disease International.

Figure 1.1. on p.53 is reproduced with kind permission of Tim Morris.

Three levels of dementia impact list (Prince *et al.* 2015) on p.95 is reproduced with kind permission of Alzheimer's Disease International.

Figure 4.2 on p.133 is reproduced with kind permission of Daisy Morris.

Action plan list on pp.149–50 is reproduced with kind permission of World Health Organization.

Core elements of self list (Bryden 2018) on p.203 is reproduced with kind permission of Jessica Kingsley Publishers. Information on the Alzheimer's Café on p.207 is reproduced with kind permission of Alzheimer Café UK.

Key elements relating to dementia cafés list (Greenwood *et al.* 2017) on p.213 is reproduced with kind permission of BMC Geriatric.

Group singing list (Clift *et al.* 2008) on p.225 is reproduced with kind permission of Sidney De Haan Research Centre.

Remember to Dance list (Vella-Burrows and Wilson 2016) on p.230 is reproduced with kind permission of Sidney De Haan Research Centre.

Promoting visual comfort and orientation list (McNair, Cunningham and Pollock 2010) on p.262 is reproduced with kind permission of Dementia Services Development Centre.

Introduction

It has been a number of years since we the authors have collaborated on exploring and expressing our observations around the lived experience of those affected by dementia and associated care approaches (Morris and Morris 2010). It has been heartening to note within the intervening years further developments in public awareness, impacted by timely campaigns and governmental policies. The communal campaigns embrace a wide variety of communicative platforms including social media and seek to promote a collective cognisance with messages of optimism and a lessening of stigma.

This book builds upon the significant theme of the 'lived experience' for people with dementia, their families, friends and significant others. It is in essence family-centred, acknowledging the experience that each family member undergoes when one family member is presented with a dementia diagnosis. For the purposes of this perspective, we introduce the readers to the Lawrence family. Each chapter takes the reader on a different part of this family's dementia journey. Their experiences are introduced through narratives that are assimilated through our examination of published sources and first-person accounts embracing 'lived experience'. This work therefore adopts a person-centred approach reflecting the concept of personhood as developed by Tom Kitwood (1997) and the Bradford Dementia Group. Our chosen family places this work predominantly within the experience of young-onset dementia and the impact upon those regarded as being in their mid-life. This provides a distinct focus concerning the 42,000 people diagnosed within the UK at younger ages (Alzheimer's Society 2019) who may well still be in employment or related areas of productivity, with families (including school age children) and active social leisure lives. Whilst this forms the predominant perspective it is intended for the reflected themes to be applicable to wider groups. This is not exclusive and we will also look at other defining characteristics including older age adults, same-sex partnerships and varying cultural groups.

Dementia (definition and statistics)

Dementia is an overall term for diseases and conditions characterized by a decline in memory, language, problem-solving and other thinking skills that affect a person's ability to perform everyday activities (Dementia Statistics Hub 2017). There are over 200 sub-types of dementia, but the five most common are: Alzheimer's disease, vascular dementia, dementia with Lewy bodies, fronto-temporal dementia and mixed dementia (Dementia UK 2019). The reader should become cognisant with other causes of dementia such as posterior cortical atrophy, Creutzfeldt-Jakob disease, dementias associated with Parkinson's disease, HIV/AIDS and alcoholism. Down's syndrome is the most common genetic cause of learning difficulties and individuals with this condition represent the largest group of people with dementia under the age of 50 years. However, cognitive assessment is challenging and diagnostic methods have not been fully validated for use with these patients and therefore early diagnosis remains difficult (Ballard *et al.* 2016).

It is estimated that worldwide approximately 50 million people have dementia with nearly 10 million being newly diagnosed each year. These numbers are estimated to increase to 152 million in 2050, a 204 per cent increase (World Health Organization 2017). In the UK there are 850,000 people with dementia with numbers set to rise to over 1 million by 2025 and 2 million by 2051. These figures account for over 42,000 people under the age of 65 and 25,000 people from black, Asian and minority ethnic (BAME) groups (Alzheimer's Society 2019). The projected increase in figures shows a continuation of a trend seen over the past few decades. From 2005/06 to 2016/17 the number of people on the dementia register rose from:

- 213,000 to 485,461 in England (increase of 115%)
- 9550 to 13,617 in Northern Ireland (increase of 43%)
- 13,234 to 19,239 in Wales (increase of 45%)
- 29,603 to 45,139 in Scotland (increase of 52.5%).

(Dementia Statistics Hub 2017)

If we take note of the sheer number of people being diagnosed with dementia we need to be mindful of the vast number of other people who are also affected. There are an estimated 21 million people in England with a close friend or family member living with dementia (Public Health England 2016).

From a cultural perspective the number of people with dementia from black, Asian and minority ethnic groups is also expected to rise significantly. The Centre for Policy on Ageing and the Runnymede Trust estimate the current number of 25,000 people with dementia from BAME communities in England and Wales to grow to nearly 50,000 by 2026 and over 172,000 people by 2051, a seven-fold increase over 40 years. It compares to just over a two-fold increase in the numbers of people with dementia across the whole UK population in the same time period (All Party Parliamentary Group on Dementia 2013).

Policy initiatives

In 2009 the then government produced the first National Dementia Strategy (*Living Well with Dementia*) that outlined three key ambitions to improve the quality of life for people with dementia and their carers in England:

- raising awareness of dementia and removing the stigma that surrounds the condition
- improving diagnosis rates for people with dementia
- increasing the range of services for people with dementia and their carers.

Some three years later Prime Minister David Cameron launched a Challenge on Dementia (*Dementia 2012: A National Challenge*) with a foreword that stated:

> Dementia is one of the biggest challenges we face today – and it is one as a society we simply cannot afford to ignore any longer. We have made some good progress over the last few years, but there is still a long way to go.

The aims were to deliver major improvements in dementia care and research in England by 2015. Three key areas were identified:

- *creating dementia-friendly communities that understand how to help* – improving awareness among the public, and the establishment of recognized dementia-friendly communities, led by the Alzheimer's Society
- *driving improvements in health and care* – including better diagnosis; improving care in hospitals; improving standards in care homes; more information for patients and families; more support for carers
- *better research* – including increased funding for research into care, cause and cure with a commitment to more than double funding for dementia research.

Also identified was a need to reduce the use of antipsychotic medication for people with dementia.

In 2015 the prime minister outlined the progress that had been achieved since the 2012 objectives:

> There has been significant progress – with more people now receiving a diagnosis of dementia than ever before, over 1 million people trained to be dementia friends to raise awareness in local communities, and over 400,000 of our NHS staff and over 100,000 social care staff trained in better supporting people with dementia. Our efforts on research have been world leading…supported by a doubling of research spending. We now spend over £60 million each year.

The document also reported that antipsychotic prescriptions for people with dementia had been reduced by 52 per cent between 2008 and 2011.

A successor, in 2015, was *The Prime Minister's Challenge on Dementia 2020* with objectives of boosting research, improving care and raising awareness about the condition in England and the following year an *Implementation Plan* with four themes:

- risk reduction
- health and care
- awareness and social action
- research.

Health provision has now become a devolved matter and to that end Scotland, Wales and Northern Ireland are responsible for setting their own policies:

- Scotland's National Dementia Strategy 2017–2020 was published in June 2017. The third national strategy maintains a focus on improving the quality of care for people living with dementia and their families through work on diagnosis, including post-diagnostic support; care co-ordination during the middle stage of dementia; end of life and palliative care; workforce development and capability; data and information; and research.
- The Welsh Government's Dementia Action Plan for Wales 2018–2022 was published in February 2018. It aims to create new ways of caring, training and increasing the number of support workers, increasing rates of diagnoses and strengthening collaborative working between social care and housing. The plan is supported by an extra £10 million a year.
- The Northern Ireland Executive's Dementia Signature Programme, Dementia Together NI, ran for four years from 2013 to 2017. It was

> jointly funded by the Executive and the Atlantic Philanthropies, under the Delivering Social Change Framework, which aims to tackle poverty and exclusion in Northern Ireland. It aimed to raise awareness, information and support for people living with dementia; deliver training and development for those in the caring professions, both formally and informally; and provide respite, short breaks and support for carers.

The All Party Parliamentary Group on Dementia (2013) emphasized the need to develop appropriate services and improve access to high quality services for people with dementia from ethnic minority groups. This report also highlighted the need for service providers to avoid stereotypes and assumptions that ethnic families 'care for their own' so do not require help.

The family

As previously mentioned, the focus within this book is upon the family, examining their individual and collective experience when one of their members is diagnosed with dementia. This family-oriented approach is heightened by the addition of first-person narratives from our constructed Lawrence family. Peter and Gill Lawrence are both in their fifties and they have three children, Ashleigh, Matt and Tom. As with subsequent chapters, you will be *invited* to accompany the Lawrence family through each distinct stage of their dementia journey, commencing at the point of first signs noted that something is wrong.

The role assumed by you is of intimate acquaintance, a family member or a long-standing friend. Travelling with them on this journey provides you with opportunities to appreciate how the condition of dementia impacts upon them individually as well as collectively. A range of activities, exercises and points of reflection are offered throughout each chapter, prompting you to consider what your thoughts and feelings are about the narrative experiences covered as well as how you might engage with those concerned. The following information contains the factual backdrop to the Lawrence family.

A snapshot of the family in the modern era is derived from the Modern Families Index (2018). The Index is the most comprehensive survey of how working families manage the balance between work and family life in the UK. Two thousand, seven hundred and sixty-one working parents across the UK responded; they each had at least one dependent child aged 13 or under. The sample comprised 1304 fathers and 1457 mothers spread equally across 12 regions of the UK including Scotland and Wales. Single-parent households accounted for 21 per cent of the sample, and married couples were the most frequently occurring at 63 per cent.

- In 2017, there were 4.94 million married or civil partner couple families with dependent children in the UK. Of the 14 million dependent children living in families, the majority (64%) of dependent children live in a married couple family (ONS 2017).
- There was strong evidence of extra working occurring, where parents said they were working beyond their contracted hours each week. The majority of respondents were contracted to work between 35 and 40 hours per week (47%), with 10 per cent contracted to work more than this and 43 per cent contracted to work below 35 hours per week.
- It is evident that for many parents working extra hours is a regular occurrence. For those parents working 'normal' full-time jobs (seven to eight hours a day, five days a week), the numbers putting in extra time is substantial. Of those parents who are contracted to work 35–36 hours per week, 40 per cent were putting in extra hours, of whom almost a third were putting in an extra seven hours (the equivalent to an extra working day) each week. Parents who work part time are also finding themselves working extra hours. For example, 34 per cent of parents who worked 25 hours per week were doing extra hours, and 30 per cent of those were putting in enough hours to qualify as full-time workers, doing around 35 hours per week.
- Working choices and working time are tied to income – the work–life choices parents would make if they had sufficient income would be different from the ones that they have to make to get by. Fifteen per cent of parents who said they have increased their working time in order to bolster their family's income also feel their work–life balance is becoming increasingly stressful.

It is worth noting that many parents (53%) expected to become carers for other adults. Of these, 22 per cent thought they would become carers within the next five years, and a further 31 per cent thought this would happen within the next decade. Those parents aged 46+ were particularly likely to identify caring as likely – 70 per cent foresaw a caring responsibility within the next ten years. Recent research carried out by the Universities of Sheffield and Birmingham suggests that two-thirds of UK adults can expect to become an unpaid carer during their lifetimes (Carers UK 2019).

The statistics above provide some of the context for families and their juggling of work and caring responsibilities. Add into the mix the presence of dementia, a condition that commonly carries such feared consequences, and we can begin to imagine that families will struggle.

Meet the family

Peter and Gill Lawrence have a close relationship and have been married for 29 years. They have three children – Ashleigh (22), married to Chris, with a two-year-old daughter, Hannah; Matt (18), a first-year university student; and Tom (11), school pupil. Peter (55) is a university history lecturer and Gill (54) is a part owner in a florist shop. Over the past year tensions in the family have been increasing with arguments taking place on a frequent basis. Gill feels exhausted most of the time, struggling to balance all her responsibilities. Peter's erratic and uncharacteristic behaviour is beginning to cause concern.

Family members

PETER

Peter's work situation has undergone some recent changes with the university being in the throes of a five-year reorganization plan, and some of his colleagues have decided to take early retirement. It is becoming an increasingly stressful place to work and Peter is struggling to cope with the increased demands and expectations. He is a member of a number of local societies and along with Gill has a fairly active social life. He is recently finding himself feeling more tired and quick to become irritable.

GILL

Gill is a partner in a small florist shop situated on the high street where they live. This last year there have been some financial problems as the result of a new supermarket being established nearby and the landlord considering raising the rent. However, the florist does generate an income for Gill and local orders continue to come in. Sometimes her uncertainties about the future spill over at home as she expresses these concerns to Peter. Gill enjoys her work and feels her independence may soon be challenged. She tries not to burden their three children with these concerns but has often told Ashleigh of her worries.

ASHLEIGH

Ashleigh is 22 years old and lives a couple of miles away with her husband Chris and two-year-old daughter, Hannah. She is aware that her mum has been concerned for some time about her dad's health…

MATT

Matt is 18 years old and is a first-year student at university in the south of England, many miles from home. For a long time he had been looking forward to leaving home and living a more independent life. What has become evident is that his trips home have become less frequent recently as he has started to fit in well with university life both socially and as a student. In a recent telephone conversation, his mum has told him about her concerns regarding his dad's behaviours.

TOM

Tom is 11 years old, lives at home and is in his final year at primary school. Last year's final school report showed a slump in subjects that he had previously gained high marks for. He appears to be concerned about the health and welfare of his mum and dad…

Early-onset dementia and mid-life

Nearly a century ago Hall (1922, p.vii) offered views on age and specifically mid-life:

> Our life is bound by birth and death, has five stages:
>
> 1. childhood
> 2. adolescence from puberty to full nubility
> 3. midlife or the prime, when we are at our apex of our aggregate of powers, ranging from twenty-five or thirty to forty or forty-five and compromising thus the fifteen or twenty years now commonly called our best
> 4. senescence, which begins in the early forties, or before for women
> 5. senecitude, the post-climacteric or old age proper.

Arguably these views pre-date the advancements achieved in subsequent decades in the fields of medicine, science, education and social change, to mention but a few. However, by the mid 1980s literature on mid-life was ushering in an increased awareness of life's finality with a suggestion that the word 'crisis' was synonymously connected with the term 'mid-life'. In fact it was in the 1960s that Elliot Jacques, a Canadian psychoanalyst (1965) coined the term 'mid-life crisis' to describe challenges during the normal period of transition and self-reflection many adults experience from age 40 to 60 years.

Cohler (1982, p.223) posited:

> A major consequence of the attainment of midlife is the recognition that more than half one's life may already have been lived... Such recognition leads to a foreshortened sense of the lifeline, and in turn, to increased awareness of mortality.

Mid-life has been defined as occurring between the ages of 40 and 65 years and is associated with periods of peak functioning including aspects of cognitive functioning, the ability to deal with multiple roles and stressors including being an employee, partner, parent and financial provider (Lachman 2004). As Peter and Gill are in their fifties and both entering their 'mid-life' it is proving an important milestone for them. As the reader you may have already arrived at this time in your life or it may be an event in the distant future. Consider what your thoughts are regarding the following questions:

- What sense do you make of the term 'mid-life'?
- Is it defined by a number?
- Is it a life stage?
- Is it an awakening that the 'best of one's life' (physically, socially and psychologically) is starting to be in the past and adaption becomes your new mantra?
- Is it a time to fight one's health concerns (physically, socially and psychologically) and 'feel comfortable' with yourself and others?
- Is it a myth?

Your answers to the questions above are likely to differ from responses that might have been made by others in previous years. Now expectations are that we will be living longer and better. We also see the retirement age gradually extending, in part as an attempt to cope with the pensions crisis but also with expectations of prolonged productivity. For families presented with a young-onset dementia diagnosis (dementia being commonly associated with advanced age) it will no doubt be a shock and, as shown by many narratives, it brings their impending mortality into sharp focus. This book is concerned with what happens to families and how they cope with the new and unexpected journey that is forced upon them by a dementia diagnosis.

Book style

This book is offered as a workbook and it is our intention that readers become actively engaged with this resource in order to maximize knowledge and understanding. The importance of this is also highlighted by the strong focus throughout upon personal narratives, and we would wish for readers to *attend* attentively to what is being expressed. In order to encourage the reader to become less of a passive recipient of other people's words and more of a reflective and active listener of their own thoughts, feelings and behaviours, we offer a series of activities and exercises.

As a starting point, please briefly consider Activity 0.1.

ACTIVITY 0.1

What are your thoughts and feelings about the term 'diagnosis of dementia'?

Reflecting on your response may have begun with a series of rhetorical questions, such as:

- What do I know and what don't I know?
- What experiences have informed my beliefs and feelings?
- How rigid and fixed are my values?

Such internal questions may have evolved over time as past and present attitudes and awareness were formed, adjusted, adapted and reformed. This often takes place countless times, influenced by our relationships and associations with peer groups, parental figures and teachers, as well as our interactions with chosen media sources.

However, your responses may also have been influenced by external rhetorical questions, such as:

- Do I know a person with dementia?
- What are my thoughts and feelings when in their company?
- What are my initial and long-term evaluations of this relationship?
- What conclusions can I draw from this?

Internal and external questioning may result in fleeting or more enduring changes that may reflect either minor reassurances about how you think and behave towards a person with dementia, or have a more pronounced influence by encouraging and challenging your beliefs and behaviours towards the person and their diagnosis.

Each chapter includes a range of reflective prompts:

- a series of activities that focus upon chapter themes intended to prompt reflection and engagement whilst reading the text
- an exercise (the full text of which is in Chapter 8) as an aid to teaching/group facilitation, which is intended to be developed or researched away from the text
- a 'How true could this be today?' section, which cites earlier writers' works and asks the reader to reflect on their significance in contemporary times.

As a point of note the 'How true could this be today?' sections are inspired by Tom Kitwood's (1997) reimagining of dementia care, which adapted and applied a humanist person-centred ethos from the earlier work of Carl Rogers and Abraham Maslow. We have accordingly selected other writers' and researchers' work that we believe can be refocused upon contemporary dementia care.

This book is structured around three distinct parts.

- Part 1 – First Experiences
  - Chapter 1 – Something's Wrong
  - Chapter 2 – Getting a Diagnosis
- Part 2 – Living with Dementia
  - Chapter 3 – Making Sense of Things
  - Chapter 4 – Commencing the Dementia Journey
  - Chapter 5 – Struggling
- Part 3 – Living Beyond Dementia
  - Chapter 6 – Coping
  - Chapter 7 – Dementia Champions
  - Chapter 8 – Exercises

As this text proposes to follow the dementia journey, some readers might look at this structure and feel that it is incomplete without additional chapters such as, perhaps, 'Seeking Residential Care' or 'Coping with Death'. The format here is intentional and we make no apologies for these omissions. Whilst further decline for those with dementia (and in a sense all of us) is inevitable we choose to pause the journey and leave the family finding ways to cope and live *beyond* their dementia diagnosis. This continuation of lives that are still there to be lived is such a powerful message that we are choosing to stop and leave the reader contemplating further upon this stage.

The chapters within this work are structured around a series of selected themes. Each theme commences with a Lawrence family narrative serving the purpose of introducing core issues and contextualizing them within a lived experience perspective. These are in essence a 'composite' of elements extracted from wider first-person narratives available within the public domain. Whilst the predominant Lawrence voice heard is that of Gill, readers are periodically granted access to the thoughts and reflections of other family members.

A summary of this book's chapters is provided here.

Part 1 – First Experiences

Chapter 1 – Something's Wrong

This chapter is concerned with the growing awareness of problems when dementia symptoms first become manifest. It details the first real awareness that something might be wrong and the processes that delay acknowledgement of what is occurring and seeking help. Initially, it is common for rationalizations to be applied that account for erratic or confused behaviour (i.e. approaching old age or stress). There are many instances where difficulties are concealed from family members giving rise to misunderstanding and tensions in relationships. The point of finally affirming that help is needed is marked by 'decisive moments' – experiences that are so noticeable they cannot be explained away. Activities, exercises and points of reflection focus upon approaches to establishing therapeutic relationships and conducting assessments.

Chapter themes:

- First signs – 'There's something wrong'
- Rationalizations – 'It'll be stress'
- Compensatory strategies – 'Whatchamacallit'
- The decisive moment – 'We need to get help'

Chapter 2 – Getting a Diagnosis

The main feature within this chapter is the process of being tested and of receiving a dementia diagnosis. This chronicles the frequent assessments, scans and tests that individuals have to endure and the terrible strain of the agonizing wait for results. For each family member or friend there will be certain worries, fantasies and expectations about what might be revealed.

The moment of receiving the diagnosis is covered in depth, illustrating the sense of shock and disbelief at what this initially means to individuals and their families, especially with young-onset dementia and the relatively young age of those concerned. The impact upon family dynamics and relationships through the testing period is examined in detail. Activities, exercises and points of reflection are geared towards promoting a greater appreciation of what is experienced and how best to support families and friends through this difficult process.

Chapter themes:

- First contact – 'Stepping into the unknown'
- Being tested – 'Waiting for news'
- The diagnostic process – 'Is it depression?'
- Receiving a diagnosis – 'It's dementia!'

Part 2 – Living with Dementia

Chapter 3 – Making Sense of Things

This chapter addresses the aftermath of receiving a dementia diagnosis. It acknowledges the bewildering process of trying to make sense of things and appreciate what the receipt of a dementia diagnosis actually means. For each family member there will be significant issues concerning the realization that 'I have dementia'; 'my partner has dementia'; 'my father has dementia'. Common feelings include a sense of disbelief, considering that the medical professionals might be mistaken, and that there could be other explanations such as undiagnosed medical conditions to account for things. Family members relate very mixed emotions at this stage including feelings of numbness and panic about the future. Core concerns including how to inform family and friends and their expected responses are covered. Activities, exercises and points of reflection are geared towards providing education, initial support and signposting to appropriate services.

Chapter themes:

- Emotional support needs – 'We are in shock'
- Implications – 'What happens to us now?'
- Initial follow-up support – 'We are in need of information'
- Making sense – 'Why me? Why us?'
- Telling others – 'Who should we tell? What can we say?'

Chapter 4 – Commencing the Dementia Journey

The issues detailed in this chapter concern the range of changes that are made by family members in order to accommodate a person with dementia's developing needs. These changes impact upon individuals in a number of ways with aspects such as financial, social and emotional implications to contend with. A family's financial stability is threatened through members having to reduce working hours or take retirement. Social contact becomes restricted through the reduction in leisure activities and difficulties encountered with others. Emotional and psychological distress is caused through numerous changes for individuals and the collective family in terms of role, status and perceptions of self. Changes can include family members taking on a caring role, something that can evoke mixed feelings and reservations. Changes in how the family perceives itself and its various dynamics are also significantly impacted upon. Activities, exercises and points of reflection are especially related to holistic support needs.

Chapter themes:

- Person with dementia: beginning the illness journey – 'I have a condition'
- Partner/carer: on becoming a carer – 'We are a couple with dementia'
- Children/family members: role transitions – 'We are a family with dementia'

Chapter 5 – Struggling

A central feature of this chapter is that of 'loss' and the influence upon personal and family dynamics. The steady deterioration of function as a consequence of dementia can have a significant impact upon individuals' sense of independence and self-esteem, for example, having to stop driving. A person's growing dependence results in others having to become more involved as *carers* and reported problems include fatigue, stress, becoming progressively detached from social and work interests and a relegation of personal needs. This evokes mixed feelings amongst carers including tension and resentment, directed towards the person being cared for or others who they perceive are not assisting as much as they could. The sense of loss is also powerfully experienced as loss of self, partner and parent. Support needs, available help and resources for individuals and the whole family are considered here. Activities, exercises and points of reflection are significantly focused upon supporting individuals around their emotional and psychological needs.

Chapter themes:

- The burden of dementia – 'It's all becoming too much'
- Identity crisis and loss of self – 'I am disappearing'
- Isolation and separateness – 'We are feeling very alone'
- Despair – 'The future looks bleak'

Part 3 – Living Beyond Dementia

Chapter 6 – Coping

This chapter provides a strong contrast to the previous chapter, illustrating ways in which individuals and their families find ways of coping and living well – despite the presence of dementia. It illustrates ways in which 'sufferer' labels are rejected by individuals with a stronger focus upon what a person with dementia can still do. Activities, exercises and points of reflection highlight approaches to supporting well-being and enhancing independence for different parties living with dementia. This chapter is strongly inspired by Kate Swaffer's (2016) timely and inspirational work.

Chapter themes:

- Living beyond dementia – 'I'm still here'
- Peer support – 'I'm not alone'
- Creative arts (self-expression and therapeutic benefits) – 'Finding my voice'

Chapter 7 – Dementia Champions

This is a different chapter in style to the preceding ones, taking a step back from the Lawrence family and exploring various ways in which dementia awareness and coping are promoted. It centres around a range of innovative projects and campaigns that are having far-reaching effects. Activities and points of reflection highlight means of supporting individuals and groups in their educational/ambassadorial role.

Chapter 8 – Exercises

Chapter 8 is devoted to structured exercises designed to explore and enhance readers' attitudes and approaches to those living with dementia.

* * *

Each chapter includes a published commentary with the heading of 'How true' (was it, is it or will it be) and asks you to reflect on your personal and/or professional experiences and understanding. We believe that the reader's age, life experiences, cultural upbringing and familial relationships will influence responses.

How true was it yesterday?

The theme of 'How true was it yesterday?' asks you to consider how observations from the past informed thinking at the time. This commentary has been chosen in order to encourage you to consider its relevance. Being mindful that hindsight can often provide a 'correct' answer to often difficult situations, your values remain important.

Background information: over two decades ago Sabat and Harré (1992) offered a description on the social construct of dementia arguing that a sense of self is still retained by the person but the public self can be lost if others fail to acknowledge it. They concluded that the attitudes and behaviours shown by other people can negate the person's sense of self if they ignore or demean it.

- What are your present-day views on this earlier social construct?
- Do you believe that these attitudes still prevail or not today?
- What personal and/or professional evidence have you for your responses?

Your age, your involvement with dementia services and your understanding of the impact this can have on the person and significant others in their life will contribute to your responses.

Concluding thoughts

We hope that this introductory chapter has effectively communicated what this book as a whole is about. It is primarily concerned with how dementia is experienced not just by the person who is presented with a diagnosis but by whole families. It traces their journey from the point of first becoming aware that something might be wrong, through the testing and diagnostic process and beyond. Whilst the main focus is upon young-onset dementia, the attention within the discussed themes is sufficiently broad to also encompass families at more advanced ages.

References

All Party Parliamentary Group on Dementia (2013). *Dementia Does Not Discriminate: The Experience of Black Asian and Minority Ethnic Communities.* Accessed on 21/2/17 at www.alzheimers.org.uk/2013-appg-report.

Alzheimer's Society (2019). *What Is Dementia?* Accessed on 24/5/19 at www.alzheimers.org.uk/about-dementia/types-dementia/what-dementia.

Ballard, C., Mobley, W., Hardy, J., Williams, G. and Corbett, A. (2016). 'Dementia in Down's syndrome.' *The Lancet Neurology 15*, 622–636.

Carers UK (2019). *Will I Care? The Likelihood of Being a Carer in Adult Life.* Accessed on 25/5/19 at www.carersuk.org/images/News__campaigns/CarersRightsDay_Nov19_FINAL.pdf.

Cohler, B. (1982). 'Personal Narratives and Life Course.' In P.B. Baltes and O.G. Brim (eds) *Life-Span Development and Behaviour* (Vol. 4). New York: Academic Press.

Dementia Statistics Hub (2017). Accessed on 21/2/18 at www.dementiastatistics.org.

Dementia UK (2019). *Understanding Dementia.* Accessed on 7/5/19 at www.dementiauk.org/understanding-dementia/what-is-dementia.

Department of Health and Social Care (2009). *Living Well with Dementia.* London: Department of Health and Social Care.

Department of Health (2012). *Prime Minister's Challenge on Dementia.* Accessed on 21/2/17 at www.gov.uk/government/news/prime-minister-s-challenge-on-dementia.

Hall, G.S. (1922). *Senescence, The Last Half of Life.* New York: D. Appleton and Company.

Jacques, E. (1965). 'Death and the mid-life crisis.' *International Journal of Psychoanalysis 46* (4), 502–514.

Kitwood, T. (1997). *Dementia Reconsidered.* Buckingham: Open University Press.

Lachman, M. (2004). 'Development in midlife.' *Annual Review of Psychology 55*, 305–331.

Modern Families Index (2018). Accessed on 21/3/17 at https://workingfamilies.org.uk/publications/mfindex2018.

Morris, G. and Morris, J. (2010). *The Dementia Care Workbook.* Buckingham: Open University Press.

Northern Ireland Executive's Dementia Signature Programme, Dementia Together NI (2017). Accessed on 2/5/18 at www.publichealth.hscni.net/sites/default/files/Dementia_newsletter_issue12_0.pdf.

ONS (2017). *Families and Households.* Accessed on 12/5/18 at www.ons.gov.uk/peoplepopulationandcommunity/birthsdeathsandmarriages/families/bulletins/familiesandhouseholds/2017.

Prime Minister's Office (2015). *Prime Minister's Challenge on Dementia 2020.* Accessed on 4/5/17 at www.gov.uk/government/publications/prime-ministers-challenge-on-dementia-2020.

Public Health England (2016). *Health Matters: Midlife Approaches to Reduce Dementia Risk.* Accessed on 4/3/20 at www.gov.uk/government/publications/health-matters-midlife-approaches-to-reduce-dementia-risk/health-matters-midlife-approaches-to-reduce-dementia-risk.

Sabat, S. and Harré, R. (1992). 'The construction and deconstruction of self in Alzheimer's disease.' *Ageing and Society 12*, 443–461.

Scottish Government (2017). *Scotland's National Dementia Strategy 2017–2020.* Accessed on 3/6/18 at www.gov.scot/publications/scotlands-national-dementia-strategy-2017-2020.

Swaffer, K. (2016). *What the Hell Happened to My Brain? Living Beyond Dementia.* London: Jessica Kingsley Publishers.

Welsh Government (2018). *Dementia Action Plan for Wales 2018–2022.* Accessed on 9/2/19 at https://gov.wales/dementia-action-plan-2018-2022.

World Health Organization (2017). *World Health Statistics 2017: Monitoring Health for the SDGs.* Accessed on 3/6/18 at www.who.int/gho/publications/world_health_statistics/2017/en.

Part 1

First Experiences

Chapter 1

Something's Wrong

Introduction

This chapter is concerned with the growing awareness of problems with daily life events when dementia symptoms first become manifest. It details the first real awareness that something might be wrong and the factors that can delay acceptance of what is occurring and seeking help. Initially, it is common for rationalizations to be applied, accounting for erratic and confused behaviour with explanations of approaching old age, illness or stress. There are many instances where difficulties are concealed from family members and acquaintances, giving rise to misunderstanding and tensions in relationships. It illustrates the growing sense of unease as well as disharmony that can affect family dynamics. The point of finally affirming that help is needed is marked by the point at which Nichols and Martindale-Adams (2006) refer to as the *decisive moment*, when difficulties have become so noticeable and apparent that they cannot be explained away.

The story so far

Peter and Gill Lawrence have a close relationship and have been married for 29 years. They have three children – Ashleigh (22), married and with a two-year-old daughter Hannah; Matt (18), university student; and Tom (11), school pupil. Peter (55) is a university history lecturer and Gill (54) is co-owner of a florist shop.

Peter's erratic and uncharacteristic behaviour is beginning to cause concern.

As you work through each chapter, we will be asking you to assume a familial relationship with the Lawrences whilst remaining mindful that your age and your cultural and life experiences may not mirror theirs.

Chapter themes

Hoppe (2017) conducted 41 qualitative interviews with seven people with early-onset dementia and 39 family members in the Netherlands between 2014 and 2015. They found collaboration taking place between people with early-onset dementia and their family members in maintaining a state of uncertainty. Various rationalisations of a temporal character were sought to explain changed behaviour. Medical support was sought at the point at which individuals' health and relationships with others were threatened.

This outlines a dynamic process of first struggling to accept the reality of what is occurring until reaching a point of crisis when help is eventually sought. The journey towards proper recognition of difficulties can be a slow and cumbersome process with many rationalizations and excuses applied. These experiences are in part derived from comments within the Lawrence family and related first-person narratives and will be examined within this chapter through the themes of:

- First signs – 'There's something wrong'
- Rationalizations – 'It'll be stress'
- Compensatory strategies – 'Whatchamacallit'
- The decisive moment – 'We need to get help'

First signs ('There's something wrong')

This initial phase concerns the first hints or signs that there could be something wrong. It covers a broad experience base with early symptoms including depression, behavioural change, neurological disorders, systematic disorders and mild cognitive impairment (Draper and Withall 2016). Clearly, this will affect many aspects of a person's daily life with impacted functioning becoming progressively more apparent. The *first signs* can include a mixture of elements including a person's thoughts, feelings and behaviours which taken individually may not be considered significant but collectively give rise to concern. If people are unaware of what is going on, there is the potential for misunderstanding and subsequent tension in relationships as erratic or distracted behaviour can be perceived as uncaring, negligent or difficult. What is apparent though is the lurking suspicion that there is something wrong, giving rise to a number of fantasies and worried thoughts. John Suchet (2010, p.iv) recounts the first inkling of his wife Bonnie being unwell after she got lost at an airport: '[I] thought the whole incident through. I couldn't make sense of it. All I knew deep down, was that it shouldn't have happened.'

The sense here is of disquiet and a feeling of unease with this acknowledgement '*deep down*' that there was something wrong.

Gill's Narrative 1.1: First signs

'We have been busy decorating the house but it is taking much longer than expected. Peter seems vague and distracted most of the time, with his mind not properly on the job. I was so annoyed and shouted at him, which resulted in Peter storming out of the house. I am feeling exhausted and just want to finish and get the house back to normal. I could rant further about how unhelpful Peter is becoming in other areas, leaving me with ever more work to do. I asked him last week to get me some items from the shop on his way home from work and he came back empty-handed. He maintained that I hadn't asked him and that it was the first he had heard about it which was simply infuriating.

This on its own wouldn't be too bad but it seems to be happening all too often recently. I am becoming increasingly worried about Peter and so is Ashleigh. He looks lost at times, restless and on edge. He also had that incident last month where he went out to the garden centre and came back hours later inexplicably saying he had got lost. I don't know whether he is especially stressed at work or maybe this is his mid-life crisis or something. He is definitely more distracted and less in the "present moment" than usual.'

- *Do you think Gill should be concerned about Peter's forgetful behaviour?*
- *If you were Ashleigh, what support could you offer your parents?*

Gill's narrative illustrates the growing tension within family relationships in relation to the experienced difficulties. Without any other explanation Peter's erratic behaviour is prone to being misunderstood or framed judgementally as, for example, obstinacy, ignorance or being uncaring. There is the sense though of worry and concern creeping in given the continuous and insidious nature of the observed problems. The sense of unease or disquiet illustrated in Gill's narrative around initial signs is echoed by a number of first-person narrative reflections. These cover certain signs and symptoms including changes in mental health states and abilities to function in activities of daily living, indicating the need for a dementia assessment. Rabin, Lyketsos and Steele (1999) identified a number of these changes, which include impact upon cognitive ability, day-to-day functioning, behaviour, and personality.

The changes identified here illustrate the breadth of the impact on a person's life. As the frequency of symptoms increase, difficulties in functioning will affect a person's relationships, occupation and many other elements of daily functioning. The following lists provide a further illustration of the initial signs and symptoms, indicative of a dementia disorder.

Early indicators of Alzheimer's disease or a related disorder include factors such as trouble with higher-level tasks; withdrawal from former hobbies and interests; forgetting or losing things; problems with reading, writing or speaking; difficulties with driving; and changes in attitude or personality (Corcoran 2009).

Ten early symptoms of dementia (Alzheimer's Disease International 2020)

- memory loss
- difficulty performing familiar tasks
- problems with language
- disorientation to time and place
- poor or decreased judgement
- problems with keeping track of things
- misplacing things
- changes in mood or behaviour
- trouble with images and spatial relationships
- withdrawal from work or social activities.

The reader is reminded that when provided with lists that identify attitudes, feelings and behaviours, their merit is in appreciation of a global and/or generalized view on the potential accumulation of symptoms. However, 'lists' fail to properly appreciate the impact upon the person and their family and friends in the present time as well as their future aspirations and decisions.

ACTIVITY 1.1

What have you learnt from the themes of 'early indicators' and 'symptoms'?

If your responses were from professional experience they would include

....

If your responses were from personal experience they would include

....

Geraldine McCarthy (2010) writes about her father's worry about where the children were, even though they had all long since grown up and left home. This stuck in her mind along with a few other puzzling moments although these were initially dismissed. The expression 'stuck in her mind' is illustrative of the nagging and persistent unease about incidents that are hard to ignore. Her narrative is symptomatic of many people's experiences whereby the first, early signs occur some years before help is finally sought (Chrisp *et al.* 2011). As Robinson *et al.* (2011) found, for some carers, the contemplation of problems being explained as *dementia* is a progressive awakening with the carer and person with dementia normalizing changes, having difficulty deciding if altered behaviour is a cause for concern. Indeed, Eustace *et al.*'s (2007) study found 29 per cent of family informants of people with dementia failing to recognize a problem with their relatives' memory in the early stages. Arno Geiger's (2013, p.19) narrative is illustrative of this: 'Our father's illness started in such a confusingly slow way that it was difficult to assign changes their true meaning… Well yes, he's acting odd at times, but didn't he always?'

This shows how the progressive changes over time can be rationalized or viewed as just part of a person's quirkiness or personality.

Another theme communicated in Gill's narrative concerns Peter's getting lost on his way to a local garden centre and being missing for hours. This event remained an unexplained occurrence for Gill and a nagging doubt. Becoming disoriented and getting lost though is commonly experienced pre-dementia diagnosis and features in a number of biographical narratives (Friel McGowin 1993; Rose 1996; Suchet 2010). The impact upon carers and family members can be one of bafflement and worry as reflected by Robinson (2010, p.80):

> I first noticed something strange in Chris's behaviour – one day when we were in our usual shopping centre he became completely disorientated. He did not know where he was or which way to go and he did not recover his mental balance till we were driving home.

Early warning signs such as this will evidently cause some disquiet and anxiety amongst those concerned. The impact upon relationships is described by Hogg (2011) in her study of ten Scottish couples with ages ranging from late-fifties to late-eighties with the anticipation of a long, difficult and bewildering journey ahead of them.

The Radio 4 (2017) programme *Diary of an Alzheimer's Sufferer* provides a striking example with Cate Latto's mother noticing worrying signs concerning her own health, which went undetected by her family and friends. Indeed, her diary extracts documenting her concerns date back over 20 years before her diagnosis of Alzheimer's: 'And now I have slipped into a no man's land, no a limbo of not remembering and what has shocked me most, not being able to write clearly. Believe me, this is a very conscious effort.'

Her daughter felt that her mother was for a long time too scared to talk about what she was experiencing to others. This is understandable, especially given her relatively young age at the time and the feared implications upon her life.

ACTIVITY 1.2

From the selection of first-person narratives:

Can you identify key words or phrases that reflect that 'something is wrong'?

Young Dementia UK provides information, support and resources for those with young-onset dementia and their families. Their website contains a number of personal stories with individuals diagnosed with young-onset dementia recounting elements of their experience including the first signs:

- Jacqui (Alzheimer's): bouts of insomnia, losing sense of what was real and passing out on a building site. She recounts waking and being left feeling disorientated and confused.
- Tracey (Alzheimer's disease and posterior cortical atrophy): experiencing frequent falls (30 times in a year). She regarded herself as always accident-prone and was told by others that she was being more of a klutz than usual.
- Valerie (Alzheimer's disease and posterior cortical atrophy): clipped the wing mirror off her car a number of times and struggled with stairs and escalators. She noticed people tutting at her in supermarkets when she couldn't work out the coins.

The apparent judgemental responses from others will likely impact negatively upon a person's confidence. Valerie's experience in the supermarket for example is likely to be very dispiriting and further impacted by the steady advancement of technology and in some cases bewildering new means of purchasing goods. With this in mind, we can imagine individuals gradually withdrawing from such activities or becoming steadily dependent upon others.

Postings on the Alzheimer's Society's Talking Point forum include multiple narratives concerning family members' memory problems and associated behaviours. Commonalities show something of the worry that is evidently experienced and the not knowing who to turn to for help or advice. These emotive messages clearly represent pleas for help, outlining the concern and fear that family members can be left with, unable to work out what is happening or explain things away. Posting concerns within a dementia discussion forum gives an indication of the direction to which one's thoughts have turned. For many people, however, such a conclusion or contemplation can take a long time to arrive at with a person's relatively young age or the feared associations connected with dementia leading various rationalizations to be applied to observed behaviour.

Helen Beaumont (2009) related her growing concerns about her husband Clive in response to critical feedback about his diminishing performance at work, his melting of a plastic cake spatula in a frying pan, losing his young son in a playground and not noticing, coming home from shopping trips with the wrong items and being sent home early from a Territorial Army exercise as a 'laughing stock'. This all concerned a man in his forties with pre-school age children, far removed from the usual stereotype and commonly considered *type* associated with dementia. We can only imagine here his wife Helen's ordeal and sense of bafflement in trying to make sense of what was happening and to be taken seriously by healthcare professionals, family and friends.

EXERCISE: HEALTH CONCERNS

This exercise asks you to explore your understanding of a person's well-being and what could necessitate a 'health concern' using an eclectic approach. (See Chapter 8.)

Rationalizations ('It'll be stress')

This section deals with the sense of unease and unsettlement experienced as early symptoms become manifest. As the warning signs continue to increase there may well be suspicions of something serious being wrong. The need to understand and make sense of these experiences can cause individuals to search for likely explanations about what is occurring with a variety of rationalizations applied. It is unsurprising to note the number of ways in which people seek to explain away or cope with erratic or worrying signs. This can mark attempts to distance themselves from the emerging fears and suspicions that may be lurking in the back of their minds. Seeking rationalizations is essentially about searching for answers, reassuring themselves and tackling emerging fears. These cover a wide spectrum from aspects that are easily acknowledged and accepted such as tiredness and stress through to those causing significant distress including contemplation of serious illness.

An example that highlights the initial search for understandable and acceptable reasons is when Helga Rohra (2016) worked as a translator, putting her initial symptoms of forgetting words down to exhaustion and an excessive workload. Similarly, Lorraine made sense of her initial symptoms as being caused by her personal home difficulties and the stress from her busy and challenging role working in a Crisis Home Treatment Acute Mental Health Team (Young Dementia UK 2019). These examples highlight the initial search for understandable and acceptable reasons, an approach that will be explored through this section in connection with the experience of various family members and their attempts at this pre-diagnostic stage to cope with worrying symptoms by assigning rational explanations.

Gill's Narrative 1.2: Rationalizations

'Things are not getting any better and Peter seems to be behaving more erratically. He is becoming more unreliable leaving me with a lot more to do. His "forgetfulness" sometimes seems as if it is deliberately put on to wind me up. Why Peter would do that when I am already feeling so stressed I don't know. I am aware that his work situation is very unsettled and that must be weighing on his mind. A number of his colleagues have taken early retirement because of this. We did have dinner with Duncan and his partner Alex recently and he related how transformed he feels, so much more relaxed and energetic. If we weren't in such a precarious financial state I would encourage Peter to leave work.

I have noticed Peter's alcohol intake increasing and he is definitely drinking more than usual. The first thing he does now when getting home is get a beer or pour himself a glass of wine. Ashleigh has told me of her worries about her father's drinking and asked me whether I think he is suffering with stress. She is also upset that he is spending less time with Hannah, the granddaughter he has always been devoted to. Tom has also complained to me about his father's unavailability whenever he approaches him for help with his homework.'

- *What do you think Gill's feelings are towards Peter and do you think her concerns are justified?*
- *What reassurances could Ashleigh offer her mother about her father's behaviour?*
- *As Ashleigh, what support could you offer Tom about the current home situation?*

Gill's narrative shows a person worried and in search of answers. Not having anything concrete to base things on and only vague unsettling notions demonstrates how easily one's thoughts can wander. Here Gill contemplates various options for explaining Peter's behaviour including tensions in their relationship, his alcohol intake or potential work stress. If she is not able to confirm or establish the cause, the range of possible explanations is liable to increase, a process likely to cause tension and unrest throughout the whole family. This is all highly significant and important to acknowledge, particularly as Hogg (2011) asserts: 'The journey from pre-diagnosis onwards can be a long road. Life must still be led to the best of an individual's ability. For some, this is a bewildering experience fraught with uncertainty.'

The words expressed here are illustrative of the tension and conflict the family will experience in attempting to maintain their normal lives, in what can be a 'long road' which is 'fraught with uncertainty'. The 'not knowing' or expressed sense of bewilderment will leave the family guessing or else misperceiving behavioural cues for elements such as indifference. Gill's narrative reflects something of the difficulty experienced by family members and the strain upon relationships at this early pre-diagnostic stage, including members feeling neglected or unloved. If those involved are not able to understand what is occurring it is likely that stress within relationships will increase along with arguments and a feeling of disharmony. A particular issue here concerns the absence of understandable information with which to reframe and understand a partner's behaviour. The behavioural changes caused through early symptoms, if not understood as part of an underlying psychopathology, can understandably impact upon relationships with potent consequences. Newman (2010, p.146), writing about his partner's dementia at the age of 52 relates: 'My first reaction to his changed behaviour was to feel that he had decided that the relationship was over, and consequently I left him.'

We can only guess here how different the outcome might have been had this couple received an earlier diagnosis. It is interesting therefore to note the sense of relief noted by some family members when finally receiving a diagnosis, having a tangible reason with which to comprehend what has been going on (Carpenter *et al.* 2008). Within a younger-onset dementia group it is understandably harder for many people to initially consider the presence of cognitive deterioration, associating this with advanced age and senility.

As seen earlier, Hoppe's (2017) research with people with early-onset dementia and their family members found individuals collaborating to maintain uncertainty in order to continue living the lives they know. The 'maintenance of uncertainty' as a means of preserving equilibrium in individuals' lives is a pertinent issue to note. Here 'not knowing' can be regarded as an attempt to stave off having to consider various outcomes, especially those regarded with trepidation and anguish. It reflects Keady and Nolan's (1995) findings with individuals actively engaging with strategies to deny personal failings and maintain a veneer of normality. Distancing themselves from explanations or reasons that include serious illness such as dementia is commonly found in relation to conditions where there is a young onset. In Gill's narrative Peter's relatively young age simply makes his behavioural cues more inexplicable and baffling with various assumptions being applied. Peter's forgetfulness outlines one of the most commonly observed early difficulties relating to dementia. It is something that individuals are initially prone to dismiss by engaging various reasons to account for a person becoming more forgetful such as tiredness, stress, overwork, anxiety, depression, physical illnesses or the side-effects of certain medications (Alzheimer's Disease International 2018). For working adults such causes may be readily grasped as potential causes. These aspects feature prominently in the Alzheimer's Society's Talking Point forum with rationalizations and reassurances frequently sought from other members: 'I'm scaring myself. It will be stress, yes?' (Alzheimer's Society 2011).

The ability to 'excuse' or explain away memory lapses will be influenced by certain factors such as the frequency of occurrence or the context within which forgetfulness is observed. In some cases, though, what is forgotten will resonate and leave behind nagging doubts even though the person may be able to function normally for some time afterwards. Jim Swift's (2010, p.40) experience concerning his wife Jan provides an example of this:

> One night we went out for a meal, and Jan suddenly asked me where we had been the previous day. We had in fact visited Venice, and had enjoyed a most memorable day out... I looked at Jan and saw the utter fear in her eyes as she

> struggled to remember this fantastic day. I told her where we had been and her face cleared as the memories came back to her. I think even at this early stage I knew that the omens were bad. I lay awake most of the night thinking of what this might mean.

As Swift indicates, 'the omens were bad', signposting his lurking feelings of dread. However, as his wife Jan's 'face cleared' and memories returned we can understand a person's desire to grasp at and hold on to normality.

ACTIVITY 1.3

From the selection of first-person narratives:

Can you identify key words or phrases that reflect 'rationalizations'?

Have you ever rationalized a person's behaviours (or your own)?

The search for alternative reasons for a person's increasingly erratic or confused behaviour can incorporate a wide variety of issues and as within Gill's narrative can include drinking, with doubts and worries surfacing around a person's alcohol intake. Behavioural signs such as unsteady gait, slurred words or confusion are commonly attributed to symptoms of intoxication. Indeed, the internal experience can be similar with a feeling of one's inner equilibrium becoming agitated or disturbed. The issue here is that a person can clearly feel unsettled where behaviour mimics signs of alcohol intoxication and indeed research findings include early behavioural signs of changes in gait (Parihar, Mahoney and Verghese 2013). A personal reflection is provided by Robert Davis (1989), diagnosed with Alzheimer's, who related feeling visually overwhelmed by the rows of goods stretching out before him in the supermarket and having to cling to the wall to keep from moving sideways. Larry Rose (1996) similarly recounts stumbling and having to cling to the backs of chairs for balance, then overhearing someone refer to him as a 'drunk'. The earlier narratives from Jacqui, Tracey and Valerie featured in the Young Dementia website highlight experiences that might all be attributed by some people as related to drinking, including frequent falls, passing out in public places or stumbling on stairs. An association with drinking is likely to impact upon a person in a variety of ways causing tension in relationships as well as evoking workplace sanctions or perhaps police involvement.

Chertkow *et al.* (2008) refer to the state between normal cognition and the onset of dementia as the 'grey zone', which can include mild cognitive impairment with no significant daily functional disability. Clearly, there will be many difficulties faced in tackling the National Dementia Strategy's (Department of Health and Social Care 2009) recommendation for early diagnosis, although working more closely with families and being alert to the potential 'warning' signs will help. The fact that there are so many ambiguous and diverse signs such as sleep disturbances (Roh *et al.* 2012) leaves the experience open to multiple explanations. There is a need to tackle the associated fear and stigma that surrounds dementia, which, as Bamford, Holley-Moore and Watson (2014) assert, can lead to many people living with uncertainty about cognitive changes for a significant period of time before seeking advice. Having a better understanding of how people can live actively and well post-diagnosis as well as the range of support available would encourage more individuals to seek help and advice at an earlier stage.

ACTIVITY 1.4

Have you noticed the media reporting of *unexplained or odd behaviours* in stigmatizing ways?

If so, can you identify the types of words and headlines used?

We are mindful that the dementia experience will apply across a range of cultural backgrounds. The All Party Parliamentary Group on Dementia's (2013) demographic profiling identified the white Irish, Indian, Pakistani and black Caribbean communities as the largest ethnic minority communities in the UK. The area of the UK with the highest black, Asian and minority ethnic population is Greater London, with significant Asian communities in the West Midlands, and the North West, extending into West Yorkshire. Historically, there has been a strong evidence base from research regarding the aetiology and progression of dementia in black and minority ethnic groups (Azam 2007; Lawrence *et al.* 2010).

ACTIVITY 1.5

Were you aware of the term 'dementia' during your adolescent years and in what context?

How would you describe your cultural upbringing?

Do you know how different cultures view the term 'dementia'?

Ethnicity and religion have been identified as factors that can influence perceptions of and attitudes towards dementia and this can also influence decision making about the care that is provided (Regan *et al.* 2013). It is striking to acknowledge the fact that there is no term for *dementia* in many South Asian languages and it is often referred to as 'not being able to remember things', 'being forgetful' or 'losing memory'. The project Meri Yaadain ('my memories'*)* found that many people from Bradford's South Asian communities were not seeking help because they had little concept of dementia and regarded memory loss as an inevitable consequence of old age. Furthermore, this initiative found that people were reluctant to seek help because of the stigma attached and the strong sense of family duty to care for older relatives (Meri Yaadain 2020).

Other cultural interpretations or explanations can be applied to initially observed behaviours and symptoms. The word 'pagal' for example occurs in a number of Indian languages and describes behaviours similar to manifestations of dementia. It can also however denote madness caused by evil spirits or previous bad actions. There are a number of different linguistic terms for describing dementia-like symptoms in both Mandarin and Cantonese but these retain negative connotations, for example the word 'Chī-dāi', the first character 'chi' translating into English as 'idiotic' or 'silly', while the character 'dai' means dull-witted. Similarly we can regard Western cultures as having similar means of characterizing a person's seemingly erratic behaviour, especially when related to those with young-onset dementia.

This section has addressed the difficulty experienced by family members in facing up to or understanding what is occurring. The many potential reasons will cause some unrest in the contemplation of each with some signs or symptoms more readily bracketed as, for example, stress or the effects of drinking. The desire to maintain a veneer of normality and keep at bay acceptance or contemplation of more serious causes will influence the adoption of compensatory strategies, which will be explored in the following section.

Compensatory strategies ('Whatchamacallit')

Attempts to keep problems concealed and maintain normality can become increasingly more difficult to maintain. Keady and Nolan (2003) suggest that strategies gradually fail and close friends and family begin to notice cognitive decline and voice their concerns. An earlier study by Keady and Nolan (1995) involved ten people with early-onset dementia and 'their family supporters' who attended a memory clinic. Their work provided a nine-stage model of dementia with early stages emphasized by components including 'slipping', involving minor lapses in memory; 'suspecting', where the frequency of incidences increases and the person suspects that there is something wrong; and 'covering up' with conscious and deliberate attempts made to compensate for difficulties and conceal them from others.

It is the process of covering up that will be examined within this section, illustrating some of the compensatory strategies employed as attempts at denying recognition of the presence of more serious causes.

Gill's Narrative 1.3: Thingamajig

'Peter is becoming less confident and spending more of his time alone. I have tried to encourage him to socialize with me although he seems reluctant to do so. We did have a couple of friends come round for coffee a short while ago but it was all rather strained. He seemed quieter than usual, rarely joining in with our conversation. When he did speak I noticed he frequently seemed to lose his train of thought. I just laughed it off and, not wanting Peter to look stupid, steered the conversation away from him. I have noticed him struggling to find the right words sometimes. What's that word he says a lot now? 'Thingamajig'. I don't really recall him saying that in the past although Hannah finds it funny.

I was also perplexed when we came back from the supermarket and he took the strangest route home. When I mentioned this to Peter he just muttered something about road works that I had no knowledge of.'

- *What conclusions do you feel Gill has arrived at regarding Peter's behaviours?*
- *If you were one of the friends who visited what support or advice could you offer Gill?*

Gill's narrative shows ways in which people attempt to 'laugh off' or explain away occurrences of memory lapses or other cognitive deficits. This can include responses which, whilst appearing far from convincing, are readily accepted by family members who are also unwilling to pursue alternative reasons. Conversational lapses, if relatively infrequent, can be plugged with all-purpose fillers such as 'whatchamacallit' and 'thingamajig' or other such versatile and all-encompassing expressions. Rationales given for erratic or unusual behaviour might also be accepted despite the implausibility of suggested explanations. The main dynamic here is the process of denial (Bender and Cheston 1997; Fernandez-Duque and Black 2007) with individuals and families unwilling to face the increasing validity of what is progressively becoming more apparent. This can also serve a 'protective' function with, for example, younger or more vulnerable family members kept at a distance from the mounting concerns. However, as shown in Svanberga, Stott and Spector's (2010) study, children, when asked to estimate when they first noticed signs of dementia, indicated a time period on average 2.5 years prior to diagnosis.

ACTIVITY 1.6

Do you think that certain types of physical ill health might cause you to deny the seriousness of the symptoms?

Based upon your response, do you feel that denial of attitudes and behaviours could be some form of defence against the reality of the symptoms?

It is interesting to note that even with mounting evidence of a dementia illness many families fail to seek appropriate medical attention (Eustace *et al.* 2007). The process of denial, not wanting to properly acknowledge and accept what is happening, applies to those experiencing the problems directly as well as family and friends. Graham (2012) describes how she, in collusion with her husband, avoided addressing their concerns:

> So for a while I came up with one crackpot explanation after another. I had a partner in this exercise of self-deception. One of the many lessons I've learned is that sufferers become very canny at patching over the holes. Questions that call for a precise answer get fudged.

The dynamic reflected here covers a *partnership of deception,* a process that can be widened to encompass whole families, with all members eager to grasp alternative and less distressing options. This illustrates just how powerful the desire for avoidance can be. The ability to make excuses or bluff one's way out of situations can be an attempt to maintain 'normality'. Robinson (2010, p.81), reflecting upon her husband Chris's behaviour, noted: 'He would pretend that he knew who people were when he hadn't a clue.'

Similarly, McQueen (2010) reflects upon her father's coping with not remembering people's names by joking about it and later insisting that he did indeed know who they were. Compensatory strategies such as these can help to maintain the illusion of normality although they delay the process of diagnosis and receiving help. This means that following diagnosis, some individuals may appear to deteriorate more rapidly when compensatory strategies become less effective (Hall *et al.* 2007). Education may play a part here and the *cognitive reserve hypothesis* suggests that highly educated individuals are initially less likely to manifest clinical symptoms of dementia as they use cognitive processing or compensatory approaches that enable them to cope better (Roe *et al.* 2007).

Jenkins and Feldman's research (2018) reveals various compensatory strategies being employed by those experiencing symptoms and their family members. Persons with undiagnosed dementia withdrew from activities where their difficulties might be revealed in order to minimize others' inconvenience and to preserve their own identity. Family carers recognized occasions where their own behaviour was adjusted to try to make life go more smoothly. This was unrecognized at the time but subsequently framed as 'thinking for two'. Family members indicated that they learnt to regulate their own behaviour to level out the 'emotional temperature' for their own sakes as well as that of the affected person. At first, they were unaware of their own adjustments and described examples of unconscious adaptation. Later, they adapted consciously and occasionally found others had done the same, for example siblings and contemporaries of the affected person dropped hints about the need to 'keep an eye on them', indicating that they had noticed problems but were perhaps protecting the person's dignity using coded messages and entreaties. A significant issue here is the desire to preserve the person's dignity and maintain 'normality'. The message 'keep an eye on them' assumes a protective role but one that does not involve healthcare personnel. This perhaps alludes to the fear of explanatory reasons such as dementia and shows how families can collude as partners in deception. This sense of collusion can engage what Gerrard (2019) refers to as finding alibis to cover conversational or behavioural lapses.

Kindell *et al.*'s (2013) study highlighted how a person's communicative ability can be enhanced through added expressive techniques to compensate for neuropsychological deficits. This included a process of enactment where what a person wanted to say was acted out or performed, enabling a greater level of meaningful communication than one's limited vocabulary alone could achieve. These findings show us how creative and resourceful people can be in dealing with some of the difficulties experienced as part of their developing dementia symptoms.

The decisive moment ('We need to get help')

Chrisp *et al.* (2012) reflect upon the often lengthy delay between first noticing symptoms of dementia and making initial contact with healthcare professionals. Key themes emerging from their study were triggers, supports and constraints. The analysis draws out the social nature of the decision to engage with the healthcare system, considering the negotiations that occur and the areas that are contested. Constraints generate delays at several points during the journey from first noticing something may be amiss to making first contact with a healthcare professional. There are certain signs and symptoms a person may be experiencing, including changes in their mental health and ability to function in activities of daily living, that indicate the need for a dementia assessment. However, as addressed above, individuals may be prone to engaging in rationalizations or compensatory behaviours in response to such behaviours unless confronted with experiences or crisis points that can no longer be explained away or avoided. This is expressively commented upon by Gerrard (2019, p.64): 'Like fog that creeps up stealthily, imperceptibly until the foghorn booms and suddenly there are dark shapes looming at you out of the shrouded darkness.'

This denotes what will be addressed in the following section as the *decisive moment.*

Gill's Narrative 1.4: We need to get help

'I can't kid myself any longer, there is something seriously wrong with Peter and we need to get help. Ashleigh phoned me this morning and asked me if we could babysit Hannah whilst she went into town which of course I was delighted about. Peter generally dotes on his granddaughter and is always pleased when she visits. As he had a lot of work to do in the garden he didn't really have much time to spend with her. Hannah seemed quite content, though, drawing at the kitchen table whilst I got on with some jobs. When Peter later came in to get some tools he asked me whether she was the neighbours' daughter. This was

very unsettling and distressing. What's wrong with him? Hannah is his own granddaughter, for heaven's sake!

When I look back, though, over the past few months there are many incidents that stand out now. These were serious issues that were staring me in the face although I must have been in denial, as were all of us within the family. We were no doubt seeking to normalize things and look for explanations that weren't too scary. I know now that I just didn't want to acknowledge the fact that Peter has a serious problem. My head is now filled with terrifying thoughts. I just can't think of a rational explanation that does not frighten me to death. There must be something very badly wrong with Peter. We can't put it off any longer, we have to make an appointment to see the doctor.'

- *Do you agree with Gill's concerns and her views on the family's behaviours?*
- *To what extent do you feel Gill is justified in considering visiting their GP?*
- *If you were Ashleigh, what help and support could you offer?*

Gill's narrative reflects upon the significant problem of misrecognizing family members, something that can occur even in early stages of dementia before a diagnosis has been confirmed. This is clearly an experience that is hard to normalize or explain away. Indeed, Michael Fassio (2009, p.40) reflects upon the occasion his mother failed to recognize her own daughter and commented: 'Who is that woman in the kitchen going around like she owns the place?'

Such incidents will cause significant distress and concern and are often recognized as *decisive moments*, the point where problems can no longer be explained away and when help is finally sought. Other common decisive moments include safety concerns and can relate to wandering behaviour, becoming lost, sustaining falls and risk issues connected with cooking or driving (Nichols and Martindale-Adams 2006). Such critical events provide families with a dramatic 'wake-up call' forcing them to address the extent of the problem (Hutchinson, Leger-Krall and Willson 1997). This provides individuals with added impetus to deal with what is being avoided. The extent of the difficulty is starkly summed up by Graham (2012):

> The terror dementia sufferers must feel is unimaginable but the techniques they use to hide their difficulties…are perfectly understandable… And you have dementia in a nutshell. The physician hesitates to name it, the sufferer denies he has it, and the carer's hair turns grey… Give Dementia time and she'll announce herself clearly enough.

What is evident here is that there are many potential factors that can delay recognition of problems and a seeking of help. Family members and friends may not recognize or understand early signs, which can be fairly subtle or explained by other reasons. As Jamieson-Craig *et al.* (2010) highlight, clinicians are in some cases reliant upon carer reports to identify early signs of dementia. The journey of Australian people with dementia and their carers was explored in the work of Speechly, Bridges-Webb and Passmore (2008) who described a timeline of changes and events such as stopping driving, needing help with daily activities and contact with healthcare professionals. Their key findings were that it took almost two years to contact a healthcare professional and approximately 2.7 years from noticing symptom onset to receiving a diagnosis.

Chrisp *et al.* (2011) reported on the delays regarding early diagnosis of 31 people living with dementia and 49 carers who attended a memory assessment centre in the UK. Their findings included the following timeline journey: 'For those who reach the point of diagnosis, the mean journey time from thinking that something may be amiss to beginning the formal process of diagnosis is around three years' (p.565).

This is all fairly alarming and is something targeted within the Department of Health's (2009) National Dementia Strategy drive for earlier detecting of dementia and pursued through educational interventions, incentivization of general practitioners and the promotion of a network of memory clinics (Iliffe and Wilcock 2017). This would help families understand what is causing difficulties and engage them with appropriate services and support. As noted above, the uncertainty and sense of unease can go on for some time, even a period of years.

John Suchet (2010, p.75) recounts how he was finally confronted with his wife Bonnie's increasingly erratic behaviour when his concerns were reaffirmed by Bonnie's son: 'His words shouldn't have hit me as hard as they did – what he said confirmed what my subconscious was telling me, but what I was, I suppose refusing to confront.' This brought to his attention a number of recollections of unexplained or unusual behaviour, things that had been in the back of his mind for some time.

Knopman, Donohue and Gutterman (2000) reflect upon the unawareness or unwillingness of caregivers to recognize memory problems until they have overwhelming evidence or critical safety concerns, indicating strong emotional barriers to acknowledging dementia. Helen Beaumont's (2009, p.30) moment of realization concerning her husband Clive's cognitive decline was expressed as:

> How could I have been so blind? Clive's behaviour was so different from earlier, and things he had always managed competently were now beyond him. The truth is that things had changed so slowly and gradually that each step seemed perfectly reasonable.

These narratives are quite startling in terms of the expressions such as 'How could I not know?' They indicate the presence of fairly irrefutable evidence yet an inability or maybe unwillingness to accept their reality.

ACTIVITY 1.7

From the selection of first-person narratives:

Can you identify key words or phrases that reflect decisive moments?

Jenkins and Feldman's (2018) findings revealed that pre-clinical signs of dementia were identifiable in retrospect. Participants' accounts resulted in four themes:

- lowered threshold of frustration – participants could relate stories in which the people they now care for had become uncharacteristically intolerant, more inclined to show their frustration
- insight and coping strategies – the ability for those with some awareness of incipient dementia to make adjustments to their activities, aiming for the best outcomes for themselves and other people
- early signs of poor memory – 'putting two and two together' and recognizing signs of memory problems and disorientation
- alarming events – increased risks, difficulties with reasoning and lack of awareness of dangers.

This qualitative study found that earlier recognition of pre-clinical dementia signs would assist individuals in planning for their future and positively impact upon their experienced social exclusion, promoting the development of 'dementia-friendly communities'. The recognition that there is a problem and taking steps to understand this can provide some soothing and reassurance. As expressed by Arno Geiger (2013, p.24) concerning his father's dementia:

> What we don't understand terrifies us most. Which is why the situation

improved for us once the signs accumulated that our father was affected by more than just forgetfulness and a lack of motivation. When everyday tasks presented him with insoluble problems, absent-mindedness could no longer be invoked as an excuse. It was impossible to keep fooling ourselves.

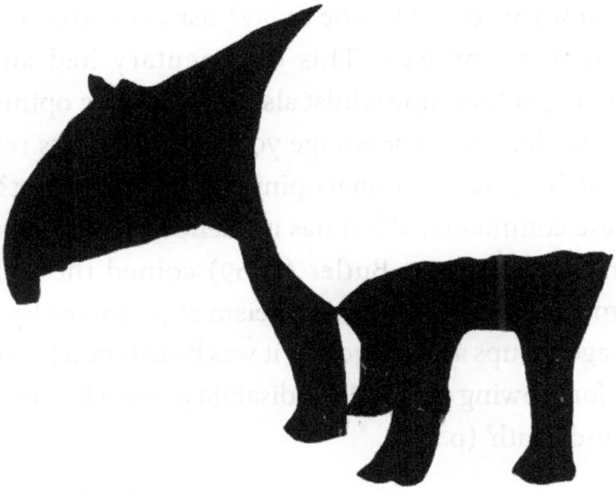

Figure 1.1 Gestalt theory and closure.
Source: Tim Morris

This narrative expresses some important elements starting with 'what we don't understand terrifies us most'. As with the Gestalt process of closure (see Figure 1.1) we are left to fill in the gaps and try to make sense of what does not make sense. The longer this process of uncertainty is maintained, the more our imagination has free rein to roam. The decisive moment alerts us to the need to seek answers and to request help. The Alzheimer's Society (2020) provide advice about seeking help:

> You should seek help without delay if your memory is not as good as it used to be and especially if you:
>
> - struggle to remember recent events, although you can easily recall things that happened in the past
> - find it hard to follow conversations or programmes on TV
> - forget the names of friends or everyday objects
> - cannot recall things you have heard, seen or read
> - notice that you repeat yourself or lose the thread of what you are saying
> - have problems thinking and reasoning
> - feel anxious, depressed or angry about your forgetfulness

- find that other people start to comment on your forgetfulness
- feel confused even when in a familiar environment.

How true could this be today?

The theme of 'How true could this be today?' asks you to consider reframing an observation from the past. This commentary had an influence in informing thinking at that time whilst also determining opinions of the day. A number of questions will encourage you to consider its relevance in the here and now, such as: have national opinions changed or not? Do you agree or not with these comments? What has influenced your attitudes?

Background information: Butler (1969) coined the term 'ageism' to describe a form of bigotry. He defined ageism as prejudice by one age group towards other age groups and suggested it was based on 'a personal revulsion to and distaste for growing old, disease, disability: and a fear of powerlessness, "uselessness" and death' (p.243).

- What are your views on this earlier observation?
- Do you believe it still exists or not in health and social care settings?
- What personal and/or professional evidence have you for your comment?
- Is there a societal tariff for a diagnosis that has no cure?

Concluding thoughts

This chapter began by inviting you to accompany Gill and her family on the first stage of their dementia journey. As a 'friend' or 'close acquaintance' of the family you have been able to access regular updates courtesy of Gill's narratives as to what was being experienced. This privileged perspective helps in getting closer to the actuality of the lived and felt experience encountered by those concerned. Hopefully this has enabled you to gain a sense of the internal world of those involved and better understand why rationalizations and compensatory strategies might be employed. Engagement with this process may have evoked in you similar feelings to those of the Lawrence family and given you encouragement to explore what you feel and think about the onset of the pre-dementia process. This provides you with opportunities to consider how you might respond to the person with dementia and their family as they strive to cope with the steady increase in erratic and unexplained behaviour from one of its members. The themes addressed here commence from the point of initial awareness and recognition of worrying signs. The sense made of what is occurring and responses made are strongly influenced by the family's homeostatic need to protect itself as an entity and maintain a sense of normality. Clearly, each person will have their own thoughts and feelings as to what is occurring as well as ways of coping with the stress and uncertainty of what might be wrong. This chapter leaves the family at the point of seeking help from healthcare professionals. The next part of the journey covers the testing process as they head towards the point of diagnosis.

PERSONAL LEARNING

What was your past knowledge and understanding, what new learning have you achieved and how could this inform your future personal and/or professional interventions?

As a 'family member', my new learning includes ....

....

On reading the first-person narratives, my new learning includes

....

INTERVENTIONS

Be mindful that whatever comments are offered should be realistic, achievable and person-centred and that the feelings conveyed and observations made reinforce that 'something is wrong' for the individual and significant other people in their life.

The types of interventions could include ....

....

References

All Party Parliamentary Group on Dementia (2013). *Dementia Does Not Discriminate: The Experience of Black Asian and Minority Ethnic Communities.* Accessed on 2/12/17 at www.alzheimers.org.uk/2013-appg-report.

Alzheimer's Disease International (2018). *Frequently Asked Questions.* Accessed on 9/4/20 at www.alz.co.uk/info/faq.

Alzheimer's Disease International (2020). *Early Symptoms.* Accessed on 1/5/20 at www.alz.co.uk/info/early-symptoms.

Alzheimer's Society (2011). Talking Point forum. Accessed on 19/3/17 at https://forum.alzheimers.org.uk/showthread.php?53803-Just-a-little-worried.

Alzheimer's Society (2012). *Dementia 2012: A National Challenge*. Accessed on 3/7/17 at www.alzheimers.org.uk/sites/default/files/migrate/downloads/alzheimers_society_dementia_2012-_full_report.pdf.

Alzheimer's Society (2020). *Short-Term Memory Problems and Dementia*. Accessed on 3/4/20 at www.alzheimers.org.uk/about-dementia/symptoms-and-diagnosis/how-dementia-progresses/short-term-memory-problems.

Azam, N. (2007). *Evaluation Report of Meri Yaadain Dementia Project*. Bradford District Health and Social Care Communication Team.

Bamford, S., Holley-Moore, G. and Watson, J. (2014). *New Perspectives and Approaches to Understanding Dementia and Stigma*. London: ILC-UK. Accessed on 17/7/17 at www.basw.co.uk/system/files/resources/basw_40614-8.pdf.

Beaumont, H. (2009). *Losing Clive to Younger Onset Dementia*. London: Jessica Kingsley Publishers.

Bender, M. and Cheston, R. (1997). 'Inhabitants of a lost kingdom: a model of the subjective experiences of dementia.' *Ageing and Society 17* (5), 513–532.

Butler. R.N. (1969). 'Age-ism: another form of bigotry.' *The Gerontologist 9*, 243–246.

Carpenter, B., Xiong, C., Porensky, E., Lee, M., Brown, P., Coats, M., Johnson, D. and Morris, J. (2008). 'Reaction to a dementia diagnosis in individuals with Alzheimer's disease and mild cognitive impairment.' *Journal of the American Geriatrics Society 56*, 405–412.

Chertkow, H., Masoud, F., Nasreddine, Z., Belleville, S., Joanette, Y., Bocti, C., Drolet, V., Kirk, J., Freedman, M. and Bergman, H. (2008). 'Diagnosis and treatment of dementia: 3. Mild cognitive impairment and cognitive impairment without dementia.' *Canadian Medical Association Journal 178* (10), 1273–1285.

Chrisp, T., Tabberer, S., Thomas, B. and Goddard, W. (2012). 'Dementia early diagnosis: triggers, supports and constraints affecting the decision to engage with the health care system.' *Aging and Mental Health 16* (5), 559–565.

Chrisp, T., Thomas, B., Goddard, W. and Owens, A. (2011). 'Dementia timeline: journeys, delays and decisions on the pathway to an early diagnosis.' *Dementia 10* (4), 555–570.

Corcoran, M. (2009). 'Screening for dementia: first signs and symptoms reported by family caregivers.' *Geriatrics and Aging 12* (10), 509–512.

Davis, R. (1989). *My Journey into Alzheimer's Disease*. Herts: Scripture Press.

Department of Health (2009). *National Dementia Strategy*. London: HMSO.

Draper, B. and Withall, A. (2016). 'Young onset dementia.' *International Medicine Journal 46* (7), 779–786.

Eustace, A., Bruce, I., Coen, R., Cunningham, C., Walsh, C., Walsh, J., Coakley, D. and Lawlor, B. (2007). 'Behavioural disturbance triggers recognition of dementia by family informants.' *International Journal of Geriatric Psychiatry 22* (6), 574–579.

Fassio, M. (2009). *Dementia and Mum – Who Really Cares?* London: Kew Bridge Press.

Fernandez-Duque, D. and Black, S. (2007). 'Metacognitive judgment and denial of deficit: evidence from frontotemporal dementia.' *Judgment and Decision Making 2* (5), 359–370.

Friel McGowin, D. (1993). *Living in the Labyrinth: A Personal Journey through the Maze of Alzheimer's*. New York: Delacorte Press.

Geiger, A. (2013). *Old King in his Exile*. München: Carl Hanser Verlag.

Gerrard, N. (2019). *What Dementia Teaches us about Love*. London: Allen Lane.

Graham, L. (2012). 'I'm Losing my Husband to a Mistress called Alzheimer's.' 27 October. Accessed on 7/8/17 at www.dailymail.co.uk/news/article-2223878/im-losing-husband-mistress-called-alzheimers-painfully-vivid-account-bestselling-novelists-struggles-living-man-coping-trials-dementia.html.

Hall, C., Derby, C., LeValley, A., Katz, M. Verghese, J., and Lipton, R.B. (2007). 'Education delays accelerated decline on a memory test in persons who develop dementia.' *Neurology 69* (17), 1657–1664.

Hogg, L. (2011). *Dementia Impact on Relationships*. Accessed on 6/5/13 at www.alz.co.uk/sites/default/files/adi-lynda-hogg-dementia-and-relationships.pdf.

Hoppe, S. (2017). 'Shifting uncertainties in pre-diagnostic trajectory of early onset dementia.' *Dementia 18* (2), 613–629.

Hutchinson, S., Leger-Krall, S. and Willson, H. (1997). Early probable Alzheimer's disease and awareness context theory.' *Social Science and Medicine 45*, 1399–1409.

Iliffe, S. and Wilcock, J. (2017). 'The UK experience of promoting dementia recognition and management in primary care.' *Zeitschrift für Gerontologie und Geriatrie 50* (2), 63–67.

Jamieson-Craig, R., Scior, K., Chan, T., Fenton, C. and Strydom, A. (2010). 'Reliance on carer reports of early symptoms of dementia among adults with intellectual disabilities.' *Journal of Policy and Practice in Intellectual Disabilities 7* (1), 34–41.

Jenkins, C. and Feldman, G. (2018). 'Recognition of preclinical signs of dementia: a qualitative study exploring the experiences of family carers and professional care assistants.' *Journal of Clinical Nursing 27* (9–10), 1931–1940.

Keady, J. and Nolan, M. (2003). 'The Dynamics of Dementia: Working Together, Working Separately, or Working Alone.' In M. Nolan, U. Lundh, G. Grant and J. Keady (eds) *Partnerships in Family Care.* Buckingham: Open University Press.

Keady, J. and Nolan, M. (1995). 'Assessing coping responses in the early stages of dementia.' *British Journal of Nursing 4* (6), 309–14.

Kindell, J., Sage, K., Keady, J. *et al.* (2013). 'Adapting to conversation with semantic dementia: using enactment as a compensatory strategy in everyday social interaction.' *International Journal of Language and Communication Disorders 48* (5), 497–450.

Knopman, D., Donohue, J. and Gutterman, E. (2000). 'Patterns of care in the early stages of Alzheimer's disease: impediments to timely diagnosis.' *Journal of the American Geriatrics Society 48* (3), 300–304.

Lawrence, V., Sams, K., Banerjee, S., Morgan, C. and Murray, J. (2010). 'Threat to valued elements of life: the experience of dementia across three ethnic groups.' *Gerontologist 51*, 39–50.

McCarthy, G. (2010). 'Back and Forth.' In L. Whitman (ed.) *Telling Tales About Dementia: Experiences of Caring*. London: Jessica Kingsley Publishers.

McQueen, I. (2010). 'Family Matters.' In L. Whitman (ed.) *Telling Tales About Dementia: Experiences of Caring*. London: Jessica Kingsley Publishers.

Meri Yaadain (2020). *My Memories.* Accessed on 2/1/20 at www.meriyaadain.co.uk.

Newman, R. (2010). 'Surely the World has Changed.' In L. Whitman (ed.) *Telling Tales About Dementia: Experiences of Caring.* London: Jessica Kingsley Publishers.

Nichols, L. and Martindale-Adams, J. (2006). 'The decisive moment: caregivers' recognition of dementia.' *The Journal of Aging and Mental Health 30* (1), 39–52.

Parihar, R., Mahoney, J., and Verghese, J. (2013). 'Relationship of gait and cognition in the elderly.' *Current Translational Geriatrics and Experimental Gerontology Reports 2* (3), 167–173.

Rabin, P., Lyketsos, C. and Steele, C. (1999). *Practical Dementia Care.* New York: Oxford University Press.

Radio 4 (2017). *Diary of an Alzheimer's Sufferer*. Accessed on 12/12/17 at www.bbc.co.uk/programmes/p0576k5t.

Regan, J., Bhattacharyya, S. Kevern, P. and Rana, T. (2013). 'A systematic review of religion and pathways to dementia care in black and minority ethnic populations.' *Mental Health, Religion and Culture 16*, 1–15.

Robinson, H. (2010). 'Glimpses of Glory on a Long, Grey Road.' In L. Whitman (ed.) *Telling Tales About Dementia: Experiences of Caring.* London: Jessica Kingsley Publishers.

Robinson, L., Gemski, A., Abley, C., Bond, J., Keady, J., Campbell, S., Samsi, K. and Manthorpe, J. (2011). 'The transition to dementia: individual and family experiences of receiving a diagnosis: a review.' *International Psychogeriatrics 23* (7), 1026–1043.

Roe, C., Xiong, C., Miller, H., Phillip, A. and Morris, J. (2007). 'Education and Alzheimer disease without dementia: support for the cognitive reserve hypothesis.' *Neurology 68* (3), 223–228.

Roh, J., Huang, Y., Bero, A., Kasten, T., Stewart, F., Bateman, R. and Holtzman, D. (2012). 'Disruption of the sleep-wake cycle and diurnal fluctuation of β-Amyloid in mice with Alzheimer's disease pathology.' *Science Translational Medicine 4* (150), 150ra122.

Rohra, H. (2016). *Dementia Activist.* London: Jessica Kingsley Publishers.

Rose, L. (1996). *Show Me the Way to Go Home.* Forest Knolls: Elder Books.

Speechly, C., Bridges-Webb, C. and Passmore, E. (2008). 'The pathway of dementia diagnosis.' *Medical Journal Australia 189* (9), 487–489.

Suchet, J. (2010). *My Bonnie.* London: Harper.

Svanberga, E., Stott, J. and Spector, A. (2010). '"Just helping": children living with a parent with young onset dementia.' *Aging and Mental Health 14* (6), 740–751.

Swift, J. (2010). 'The Departing Light.' In L. Whitman (ed.) *Telling Tales About Dementia: Experiences of Caring*. London: Jessica Kingsley Publishers.

Young Dementia UK (2019). Personal stories. Accessed on 8/9/19 at www.youngdementiauk.org.

Chapter 2

Getting a Diagnosis

Introduction

The main feature within this chapter is the experience of undergoing tests and the powerful emotions this can evoke for those concerned. Allied to this are the fears and distress experienced by family members enduring a 'barrage' of assessments, scans and tests with an understandably agonizing wait for results. As Lian *et al.* (2017) found, people with dementia and their caregivers engage in their own unique journeys as they progress towards the point of diagnosis. The sense of shock and disbelief at what a dementia diagnosis signifies for the whole family group is examined, particularly in the case of young-onset dementia, often viewed with incredulity at what was formerly thought of as 'an old person's disease'. Narratives are cited to illustrate the unique experiences that the assessment and diagnostic processes can provoke. The reader is reminded of Peter's age and views on young-onset dementia are explored.

> ***The story so far***
>
> *The previous chapter followed the Lawrence family through their struggles with the early manifestations of Peter's dementia symptoms. The early observed signs were met with concern yet passed off as indications of stress, approaching older age, overwork, drinking and other plausible causes. The increasing manifestations caused tensions and stress, impacting upon relationships in the family. The attempts to rationalize symptoms or engage compensatory strategies were eventually starkly challenged by a 'decisive moment', when Peter failed to recognize his granddaughter. This forced the family to finally relook at all of the disturbing 'incidents' that they had experienced and acknowledge that they now needed to seek help.*

Chapter themes

Campbell *et al.*'s (2016) study illustrated a four-phase sequential model relating to the diagnostic transition. This progressed through phases of becoming self-aware and seeking assistance; being referred; undergoing tests and learning what might be wrong; and finally, adjusting to one's diagnosis and facing renewed expectations.

They identified a core category of 'living with uncertainty', which ran through each stage and summarized the entire diagnostic journey for all study participants. Reflections upon this model have provided the base for this chapter's themes, which centre around:

- First contact – 'Stepping into the unknown'
- Being tested – 'Waiting for news'
- The diagnostic process – 'Is it depression?'
- Receiving a diagnosis – 'It's dementia!'

First contact ('Stepping into the unknown')

This first contact with healthcare services may feel like a step into the unknown for families, not really knowing what to expect with the emotional polarities of wanting support versus worries about what they might be told. Questions needing answers are likely to be vague or uninformed with reliance upon healthcare professionals for guidance. The need to seek help, as prompted by a 'decisive moment', covered in the previous chapter, can cause family members a dilemma between caring and coercion if there is reluctance or fear about visiting the doctor.

Gill's Narrative 2.1: First contact

'Well, today's meeting with the GP was frustrating and I'm not sure how helpful it was. I have a nagging doubt that the problem hasn't really been addressed. The doctor asked Peter a lot of questions and carried out a physical examination. He even took some blood to send off to the laboratory for testing.

"What are you looking for, Doctor?"

"Well, it's too early to say, although the symptoms your husband has been experiencing could also be explained by maybe an infection. We will need to arrange further tests and assessments."

I left with few conclusive answers. We struggled, not really knowing what to ask and it would have helped for us to have been better prepared. A couple of leaflets about coping with stress were given to us along with details of a "useful" website. We thanked the doctor but left the surgery downcast with neither of us willing to break the silence and voice our disappointment or disillusionment to each other.

We were given a further appointment to return at the end of the week when the blood results would be ready.'

- *What mixed emotions could Gill be feeling following this first meeting?*
- *If you were Ashleigh, Tom or Matt, what might you want to ask or say to Mum and Dad after their visit to the doctor?*

Gill's narrative illustrates something of the frustration and disappointment that families can experience after finally having sought medical help. It is understandable that individuals at this stage will be in need of answers as well as hoping that they can be supported with the difficulties experienced. Instead, receiving few answers and being given the indication that this is going to be a long and arduous process can be enormously dispiriting and disappointing. Gill highlights the uncertainty she and Peter had regarding what to expect and that they had no real way of preparing for this initial visit. As a consequence they felt lost when offered the opportunity to ask questions. Whilst a number of those at younger ages might not even contemplate the presence of dementia, for those that do there are various guides and resources assisting with this first contact. The Alzheimer's Society Canada (2018), for example, provides some useful advice on preparing for the initial practitioner's visit, focusing upon the stages before, during and after the consultation. Preparatory guidance suggests individuals take note of observed symptoms, list medication being taken and detail personal medical history. It also helpfully outlines suggested questions individuals might want to ask at their consultation. During the appointment they are advised to give specific examples of their concerns, take their own notes and request further explanations and clarification, including written information. On their return home, the advice urges that people review their notes, start a journal and consult with family and friends.

This very helpful guide enables families to take some charge within this process and combat some of the frustration and helplessness felt. As the testing and assessment journey is likely to be lengthy and arduous there is a need for practitioners to ensure that families are suitably prepared for each of their subsequent consultations. In the UK, carers and family members are advised by the Alzheimer's Society to accompany their relative to consultations to provide them with support and, following appointments, to help them in recalling what has been discussed. This is the guidance provided by the Alzheimer's Association (2019) when visiting the doctor.

What to bring to a visit for memory loss:

- a list of symptoms, when they began, and how frequently they occur
- a list of past and current medical problems: tell your doctor if other family members had illnesses that caused memory problems
- all medications, both over-the-counter (e.g. vitamins, aspirin) and prescription.

Be prepared to answer the doctor's questions honestly and to the best of your ability.

Questions to ask about testing for memory loss:

- What tests will be performed?
- What does each test involve?
- How long will the tests take?
- How long will it take to learn results?

Furthermore, the Alzheimer's Association's website provides a range of information plus an interactive tour that leads individuals through the various tests used.

ACTIVITY 2.1

What is your understanding of the term 'memory loss'?

Briefly consider how memory loss could influence a person's health and well-being.

Familial dynamics can become a problem when the need to seek help is not agreed upon by all the parties. The previous chapter considered 'decisive moments' that necessitate seeking help. Often these concerns are expressed by loved ones rather than the person exhibiting erratic or worrying behaviours. The Alzheimer's Society (2019a) suggest ways for family members to raise their concerns with questions to consider as well as thoughts around choosing a non-threatening place and having sufficient time for the conversation to take place. Where the person concerned still disagrees or is unable to appreciate what is occurring for them, they may not concur with the need to visit their GP. In such instances Dementia Australia (2019) urge family and friends to find different reasons such as routine physical check-ups to encourage individuals to see their doctor. Such an approach is also advocated within the UCL Department of Mental Health Services' (2005) factsheet recommending using an appointment with the GP about a separate issue, either for oneself or one's relative, to bring up the observed problems.

ACTIVITY 2.2

What are your views about these different approaches?

The approaches being suggested here can be seen as good advice or conversely felt as unsettling and deceiving by families as well as being regarded as unethical by practitioners. These competing and conflicted opinions are shown within various online discussion forums such as the Alzheimer's Society's Talking Point. An example of this concerns a discussion thread requesting help for an aged father who is reluctant to visit the doctor. The responses and ensuing discussion echoed some of the suggestions indicated above with a range of potential reasons to get him to visit their GP on another pretext such as annual health checks, medication reviews, consultation for other medical conditions, flu jabs or required visits to stay on the doctor's books. Further 'subterfuge' was noted with one respondent asking friends to call her mother pretending to be the doctor's receptionist and informing her of a booked annual health review. People clearly had very different experiences with their GPs with some less willing to accommodate such requests. Advice was given in these instances to seek a more sympathetic practitioner although one respondent found persistence and perseverance working with their GP finally getting fed up with them calling daily and offering an appointment.

This first visit marks the commencement of the diagnostic process and the next stage in what may have already been a lengthy experience, especially considering the average times varying from 8 to 52 months from first symptoms to a first encounter with a health professional (Perry-Young *et al.* 2018). The experience of being tested is covered in the following section.

Being tested ('Waiting for news')

Regardless of your age, being tested can bring back earlier thoughts and feelings, for example, when at school, in your career or taking a driving test, where results determined the degree of success or failure. For a person experiencing cognitive difficulties one can only wonder how magnified such feelings could become. Keith Oliver (2019), diagnosed with Alzheimer's in his fifties, recalls being subjected to a seemingly endless number of tests with each subsequent assessment providing a new piece in a jigsaw, with a picture gradually emerging of what his problems were caused by. The testing process was at times experienced as very dispiriting, especially being told that his cognitive test scores placed him in the bottom fifth percentile of the population:

> I had not been referred to as average since my secondary school days in French and as for being in the bottom 5 percent of anything cognitive, that is a totally new and alien feeling...going into these tests I really wanted to score as high as I could so that they would tell me at the end of the day it wasn't Alzheimer's. (Oliver 2019, p.52)

This personal reflection shows something of the lurking fear that individuals can experience along with a sense of dread that is strengthened through each subsequent test. It is also similarly felt by family members as shown by Helen Beaumont (2009) recounting the awful sensation she had when observing the distress of the physician testing her 45-year-old husband Clive and her realization that the tests were not going well. On reading the above reflections we can imagine something of the sinking feeling felt by those being assessed and their family members when it becomes clear that individuals are faring poorly with the testing process. Consider then how they might feel when this is repeated over subsequent assessments with the true extent of a person's cognitive deterioration gradually being revealed. This is all the more arduous and distressing given the time span involved with a diagnostic process that can cover several years with visits to a large number of physicians (Teel and Carson 2005). This section explores what individuals and their families experience and feel at the various stages of this assessment process.

Gill's Narrative 2.2: Testing

'We had a phone call late this afternoon from the doctor's surgery asking if we could attend the following morning. When I took the call I felt a sudden chill, caused no doubt by the sudden realization that we might hear something definite. The conversation went something like this:

"Can you tell me please what he wants to speak with us about?"

"I'm sorry I can't give you any details although I believe he wants to discuss the ongoing tests that have been carried out."

I wasn't at all impressed by this. As well as not telling us anything they have also raised our concerns. Ashleigh is convinced that it is something to worry about because of the urgency. What is especially hard about these appointments and waiting for news is in not knowing what to tell the family.'

- *Prior to this appointment, what support could you offer Gill?*
- *During this time, what support could Ashleigh offer her dad?*

Gill's narrative reflects how envisioned fears can be stimulated through each new test Peter is required to undergo. Figure 2.1 shows the polarities of 'ifs' and 'unknowns' in a diagram; you may wish to add your own views.

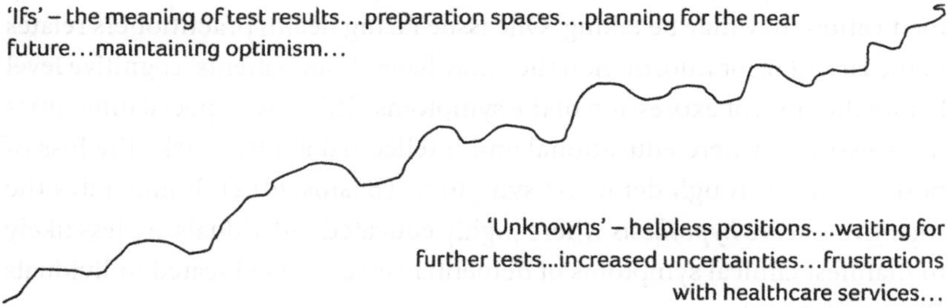
'Ifs' – the meaning of test results…preparation spaces…planning for the near future…maintaining optimism…
'Unknowns' – helpless positions…waiting for further tests...increased uncertainties…frustrations with healthcare services…

Figure 2.1 Envisioned fears

Figure 2.1 is somewhat devoid of the 'felt experience'; however, arriving at a diagnosis requires a combination of physical and psychological tests and assessments over a period of time. Unsurprisingly, undergoing the varied assessments can feel overwhelming. Davis (1989, p.58) recalls: '[being] tested by virtually every test possible. I was CAT scanned, X-Rayed, MRI scanned and every type of body fluid was tested and retested. Still nothing definitive was found.'

This indicates something of the extensive range and scope of tests used. It is a detailed process that is undertaken by a GP, a specialist practitioner at a memory clinic or a designated hospital department and involves:

- history taking
- cognitive assessment
- physical examination
- brain scan.

EXERCISE: ON BEING TESTED

This exercise asks you to consider your 'felt experiences' when undertaking formal tests or examinations. (See Chapter 8.)

History taking

History taking is a central tenet of discovering what the person is experiencing, the sense they are making of these experiences and what impact this could be having on other people. Within these conversations the practitioner will check if there are any existing conditions the person has (for example, diabetes, heart disease, depression or a stroke) and any medication they may be taking. One issue facing health practitioners relates to the lack of prior information they may have about patients' cognitive level before the current expression of the symptoms. This poses special difficulties in assessment where educational and intellectual ability masks the loss of performance through dementia symptoms (Bastos 2012). It illustrates the *cognitive reserve hypothesis* where highly educated individuals are less likely to manifest clinical symptoms of dementia versus less-educated individuals (Roe *et al.* 2007).

The value in including family members in assessments is highlighted by a Healthtalk (n.d.) interviewee who described clear discrepancies between his wife's reporting of events and his own experience.

> On several occasions when my wife was being asked questions, questions which the person answering wouldn't know whether they were right or wrong…for example, they were asking my wife if she had sex and she said 'Yes, regularly.' I knew full well that we hadn't had any sex for a number of years. I knew it was the wrong answer. But the person asking the questions wouldn't know that it was a right or wrong answer.

This interviewee subsequently made a recommendation for carers to be routinely consulted in order to get a clearer level of understanding and to facilitate the diagnostic process. This suggestion is a valid one but also suggests a need for being extended to the wider family in order to better contextualize and understand what is being experienced and the support needs of each party. The example does raise some interesting considerations that can be influenced by perceptual differences between partners. Irrespective of memory problems, couples can strongly dispute whether or not they have sex *frequently* or *rarely*. The serious learning from this is that recollections can vary and whilst we should take every opportunity to involve family members this should not mean that we disregard what those being tested are telling us. Carers and family members, though, can, importantly, help practitioners understand more about a person's prior level of functioning, as shown by Jamieson-Craig *et al.*'s (2010) research. Indeed, retrospective carer reports of changes in everyday function and memory provide important indicators of dementia.

Cognitive assessment

A second tenet to the diagnostic process is for the person to undertake cognitive assessments. These tests assess the person's mental abilities and include their short- and long-term memory, concentration and attention span, language and communication skills, as well as their orientation to time and space. A point of consideration for practitioners whilst undertaking these 'testing activities' relates to the person's level of education or language ability, as this may have an influence on the scores they achieve. For example, a person who cannot read or write very well or for whom English is not their first language may score poorly but without signposting that they have dementia.

Arguably the stress of undertaking an assessment can provide the person with the motivation and to some extent the means of proving what they know (or do not). However, the assessment process and fear of failure can cause anxiety-provoking feelings and thereby negatively impact upon attention and concentration. Such tests assume that the person being assessed has the ability to hear reasonably well, can read and write, and is able to subtract numbers in a methodical way that provides a measure of concentration.

ACTIVITY 2.3

What feelings, thoughts and behaviours could a person be experiencing during their first assessment?

If you were a health practitioner how might you engage with the person at this time?

If the person appeared worried, I would............................

If the person appeared upset, I would.............................

If the person appeared angry, I would.............................

Included below are a few of the increasing bank of assessments that seek to evaluate a person's cognitive abilities. This is by no means the definitive range although their inclusion highlights the types of questions, time scales, scoring ratios and results included. The ways these tests are delivered and an appreciation of how they might be received are commented upon, showing consideration of influences upon the person's performance and their relationship with the practitioner.

- *Abbreviated Mental Test Score (AMTS)* – incorporates ten questions with one mark for each correct answer. This largely measures a person's memory and concentration and is used for screening when a person is in hospital. An address is given, to be recalled at the end of the test. Sample questions ask about age, time (to the nearest hour) and the name of the present monarch (Qureshi and Hodkinson 1974).
- *Mini Mental State Examination (MMSE)* – this brief test (12–20 minutes) can make an initial assessment possible by measuring cognitive function (Folstein *et al.* 1975). Whalley and Breitner (2002) argue that the MMSE provides a reliable index of dementia severity and staging when used with other clinical measures. It is scored out of 30. A score of 20–26 indicates mild cognitive impairment, 10–20 moderate impairment, and less than 10 severe impairment.
- *Montreal Cognitive Assessment (MoCA)* – takes approximately ten minutes to complete. It has a maximum score of 30, with a score of 25 or under indicating the need for further assessment. It is especially helpful in assessing people with vascular dementia (Nasreddine *et al.* 2005).
- *6-item Cognitive Impairment Test (6-CIT) Kingshill Version 2000* – developed in 1983, this test consists of a logical memory item, two attention items and three orientation items. The test uses an inverse scoring system with a total score out of 28. Scores of 0 to 7 are considered normal and 8 or more significant. Sample questions include 'What year is it?' and 'Count backwards from 20 to 1' (Brooke and Bullock 1999).
- *The General Practitioner Assessment of Cognition (GPCOG)* – takes about ten minutes to complete and comprises two parts with separate questions asked of patients and carers. It contains cognitive tests and elements of history with sample questions such as recall of a notable name and address, what the date is, clock drawing and recall of recent news events. A combined score is out of 15 (Brodaty *et al.* 2002).

The tests highlighted above have a number of similar features including information recall, counting backwards and questions around orientation.

Clock drawing tests are often used, taking on average a couple of minutes to administer, and reflect frontal and temporoparietal functioning (Shulman *et al.* 1986). The National Institute for Health and Care Excellence (2018) (clinical guideline NG97) provides guidance on ways of interpreting the person's scores, and this should take full account of factors known to affect their performance including educational level and practical skills, a person's former level of functioning, language ability and sensory impediments, as well as any psychological or physical problems.

Approaches engaged in by family members, fearful about a person's performance in a cognitive test, were highlighted by Gofton and Weaver (2006) who found evidence of coaching by caregivers during the MMSE. The desire to compensate for a person's deficits can be regarded as a form of denial or desire to avoid the stark reality of what appears to be happening within the family. Assisting a person with their cognitive tests can relate to the desire to avoid or delay certain unwanted outcomes such as a discontinuation of medication or reaching the point of needing to contemplate residential care. This was illustrated very vividly within the BBC (2006) documentary *One Life: My Life on a Post It Note* about Christine Lyall-Grant, former literary editor at Cambridge University Press. This intelligent and engaging woman with young-onset dementia was prompted by her daughter to revise and prepare for her test by reciting a range of words beginning with the letter P. The daughter's concern and stressed resignation during this process is clearly visible as her mother recites such examples as plebiscite, posterior, plumage and population.

ACTIVITY 2.4

Reflect on how you felt and thought the last time you undertook an examination or test (be it physical, social or psychological).

Were you satisfied with your responses?

Were you satisfied with the way this assessment was conducted and would you change anything about it?

Arguably, when formal tests or examinations are undertaken, the outcome will consider a number of factors unique to the person being assessed:

- providing evidence of what you know and do not know
- showing the degree of your memory recall

- gauging your range of knowledge and understanding
- evaluating the ability to take control of your feelings at this 'assessment' time.

In relation to interpretation of scores and answers given, it is important that practitioners accommodate cultural factors as highlighted by Diana Harris in relation to her husband Eugene's cognitive assessment (Alzheimer's Society 2019b). As Eugene was originally from the Caribbean island of Saint Kitts she argued that his performance could well be affected when 'He was asked to recognise different types of gate, but because Eugene spent his early life abroad, his memories might be different. He may not have known different farm gates and garden gates.'

Whilst she was reassured that the consultant had a lot of experience with patients from the Caribbean it does not necessarily mean that the subtleties of cultural comprehension are recognized.

Physical examination

A third tenet involves excluding any physical causes or factors that could become confused with a diagnosis of dementia. In most cases blood tests will check the person's function levels (kidney, liver and thyroid), haemoglobin A1c (for diabetes), vitamin B12 and folate levels. Patients who have mild cognitive impairment (objective cognitive loss not affecting function and daily living activities) are routinely followed up in primary care, and if symptoms become more severe, re-referred for specialist assessment (Robinson *et al.* 2015).

Brain scan

A further level of diagnostic assessment is provided by a brain scan, which provides further evidence that could explain the person's symptoms. A magnetic resonance imaging (MRI) scan produces detailed images and can help confirm that the person has a diagnosis of dementia. It provides information about blood vessel damage (vascular dementia) and shrinkage of the brain in frontal and temporal lobe areas (fronto-temporal dementia/ Alzheimer's disease). A computerized tomography (CT or CAT) scan uses X-rays and a computer to create detailed images and check for signs of a stroke or brain tumour. A positron emission tomography (PET) scan produces three-dimensional images showing any abnormalities with blood flow in the brain (NHS 2017).

ACTIVITY 2.5

What thoughts and feelings have you experienced when waiting for a result after:

- **a medical test?**
- **an academic examination?**
- **an interview?**

In Samsi *et al.*'s (2014) study, feelings of confusion, uncertainty and anxiety over interminable waiting times dominated. Participants often felt without support to manage their uncertainties and emotions, not knowing where to turn for assistance. The wait for confirmation can be a fraught and distressing process with many fantasies and worries generated. Dillon (2016) found that this can involve feelings of depression as well as *anticipatory grief* relating to projected losses and changes in family roles. As Ross (2009) confirms, anticipatory grief is a real phenomenon that affects many family caregivers of dementia patients. Here dementia caregivers are not experiencing 'typical' grief but something much more complicated.

The diagnostic process (and misdiagnosis) ('Is it depression?')

Differing emotions and experiences can result from this first contact as the person's diagnostic process commences. For practitioners this poses a number of difficulties because various symptoms can be misleading or confirming of a diagnosis. In the early stages of young-onset dementia it is not uncommon to have symptoms attributed to other mental health conditions such as depression and anxiety. Practitioners also report their dilemma around who to tell when giving a dementia diagnosis with various justifications applied such as worries about a person's reaction or doubts over their capacity to understand.

Gill's Narrative 2.3: It's depression

'Today was the latest in our seemingly endless visits to see one medical practitioner or other. We have now been informed that Peter has depression and prescribed antidepressant medication. The doctor did say that they would continue to do more tests although she was fairly confident that Peter's stressful

work situation, level of alcohol consumption, feelings of tiredness and the tension within our relationship could all point towards a state of depression. We have also been given yet more leaflets and websites to visit including information about couples therapy. Peter has three months' sick leave from work.

I am not sure whether to feel relief or despair at this news. Depression? I felt comforted as well as unsettled to hear that they are running more tests. Could Peter have a medical condition, a brain tumour, an infection or something else? At least we have some sort of explanation to tell the family as they are all naturally very worried.'

- *What mixed emotions do you think Gill could be experiencing about this diagnosis?*
- *If you were Gill, what would you wish to say to the children?*
- *If you were Peter, what might your thoughts and feelings be about taking sick leave?*

Gill's narrative shows the mixed emotions between relief and despair at hearing Peter being diagnosed with depression. There is still a nagging doubt that there could be something else behind his symptoms including a yet undiagnosed underlying medical condition. This illustrates the complexity for practitioners at arriving at a diagnosis especially given Peter's young age and the perceived likelihood of symptoms being explained by other conditions. Before being confirmed by brain scan (i.e. CAT or PET) it is not uncommon for symptoms to be attributed to other physical and mental health causations, especially where evidence appears to corroborate this.

Chris Carling (2012) relates her father initially being diagnosed with depression and progressively given increasing doses of antidepressants before some time later receiving a diagnosis of dementia. The mimicking of a depressive episode can sometimes be referred to as depressive pseudo-dementia (Gainotti and Marra 1994). Conversely, where a person has depression (including a loss of interest and pleasure in daily activities, social withdrawal, sleep and appetite disturbances) and cognitive symptoms (including difficulties in thinking clearly, problems concentrating and difficulties in making decisions) they may appear to exhibit signs and symptoms of dementia. There is a need to consider the distinguishing features between a person with a depressive illness and a person with dementia. Brown and Hillam (2004) highlight certain distinctions with the onset of depression being more typically rapid and with identifiable triggers, whereas with dementia the underlying factors can be less determinable and the progression being more progressive. They also noted a difference with symptoms appearing worse in the morning for depression and the evening for dementia.

The Facing Dementia Survey (Bond *et al.* 2005) was conducted with more than 2500 people across Europe and sought to assess awareness and behaviours surrounding Alzheimer's disease. The sample included 618 carers (mostly spouses and children), 1200 members of the public (over the age of 18 years), 605 physicians (general practitioners), and 96 people with Alzheimer's disease. One of the key messages that emerged from the survey was that Alzheimer's disease remains undiagnosed until symptoms become moderate to severe and this may be because of the difficulties in recognizing the early symptoms and the attributions of symptoms associated with normal ageing. Moreover, delays can be influenced by the fear dementia holds for people and is often compounded by inadequate screening tools employed by physicians.

Christine Bryden's (2005, p.17) experience is illustrative of the fuzzy distinction that exists between dementia and depression:

> I had really deteriorated, changing as a person, losing the super-fast, super-smart me. I had become much slower in my speech, less able to make decisions, and more readily confused... I was well into my journey with the disease [dementia], experiencing most of the cognitive, behavioural and neurological signs of mild to moderate dementia. I no longer drove, answered the phone or watched TV, but retreated into gardening and books, as well as early bedtimes.

From the narrative here it is easy to make the assumption that her steady decline is an expected consequence regarding her Alzheimer's disease. This picture changed though as her mood improved:

> My head began to clear of the fuzzy 'cotton wool' type of feeling that it felt like before. I could concentrate better, and found it easier to speak and listen... I began to speak on the phone again, and even to start driving again. (Bryden 2005, p.18)

This experience is reflected by others' narratives who observe a number of alternative diagnoses being given before eventually having dementia confirmed (Houchen 2010). The symptoms a person experiences can provide us with indications or warning signs of presenting or impending physiological, psychological or social difficulties. However, the overlap between various ill-health states will provide a confusing and difficult picture around which to navigate. It is not surprising that the initial problems caused through a developing cognitive dysfunction will impact upon a person's self-belief system and affect their worth, esteem and awareness.

The early diagnosis of dementia is significant as it may allow both family and friends time to adapt and consider planning for the future with the person and their diagnosis in a collaborative way. Indeed the National Dementia Strategy (Department of Health 2009) advocates practices that encourage early diagnosis and support. Delaying the diagnosis can lead to lost opportunities for the person with dementia and their relatives to become included with decision-making. A point of note for practitioners concerns the uncertainty or trepidation in respect of presenting a dementia diagnosis. In the late 1990s, several studies suggested that people with dementia had definite views about being told their diagnosis including the feeling that sharing a diagnosis offered the opportunity for the person to express their fears, gather information about dementia and discuss the nature and prognosis of the illness (Husband 1999; Marzanski 2000). Overall, evidence suggests that most patients wished to be told their diagnosis and only a small number do not. For the majority who wish to know, diagnosis sharing plays a pivotal role in facilitating a focus on the experience of the person with dementia during both the early stages and throughout the trajectory of the illness; in other words, it has the potential to positively influence the approach to care and treatment in both the short and long term (Wilkinson and Milne 2003).

The effect of being told the diagnosis of dementia from the perspective of the person with dementia is outlined in the Tell Me the Truth study (Pratt and Wilkinson 2001). As part of a programme of research exploring dementia care, the Mental Health Foundation funded a project exploring the issues of diagnosis sharing from the perspective of the person with dementia. This study aimed to build on existing evidence and involved in-depth interviews with 24 people with dementia. The interviews focused on ascertaining the person's views and experiences shortly after receiving their diagnosis and explored how patients felt about the way in which they were told the diagnosis, any opportunities, and limitations associated with receiving an early diagnosis and their views on 'best practice' in diagnosis sharing (Pratt 2002; Pratt and Wilkinson 2003). Some examples of poor practice were highlighted by study participants: not being given enough information, having insufficient follow-up and being given contradictory information from different health professionals. There were some very definite views expressed about whether or not individuals should be informed: 'I would shoot the person that tried to keep it back from me…if you want to ignore it, ignore it if you wish, but it's your choice, it's not the doctor's choice, or the carer's choice' (Jack).

There can be a number of reasons, however, why detection of dementia takes place at later stages with obstacles including attitudinal factors.

Ahmad *et al.*'s (2010) work highlighted dementia diagnoses often being delayed within primary care. Whilst they found older GPs being more confident in diagnosing and giving advice about dementia, they were less likely to feel that early diagnosis was beneficial, critically perceiving patients with dementia as a potential drain on resources with little positive outcome. Younger GPs, however, were more positive and felt that much could be done to improve quality of life. A delay in diagnosing can also be made for more constructive reasons as shown in Dhedhi, Swinglehurst and Russell's (2014) study. This outlines that the reluctance, or failure, of a GP in making a diagnosis on a particular occasion need not reflect their lack of awareness around policies advocating earlier diagnosis. Instead, as they argue, it can reflect the range of nuanced balancing judgements employed with patients and their families. In these instances 'rightness' of time is favoured over concerns for early diagnosis.

ACTIVITY 2.6

As a practitioner – when would be the 'best' time to offer a diagnosis?

As a person – when would be the 'best' time to receive a diagnosis?

What would influence you arriving at the 'best' time?

Receiving a diagnosis ('It's dementia!')

The receipt of a dementia diagnosis is an impactful and momentous occasion that is associated with some extremely polarized reactions. This was shown in Husband's (1999) study concerning the psychological consequences of learning a diagnosis of dementia. Whilst one participant (Vera) reported feeling less anxious once a diagnosis was made: 'At least I know what it is, I'm not imagining it and I know what I'm facing', another (John) had a typically negative view of dementia and wanted to know how soon he would 'become a vegetable'. Burns (2012) provides a reminder on the perceptions that can envelop the question of 'what is preventing people from receiving a timely diagnosis?' He argues that there are barriers conjured in society that may be part of the answer. These include the stigma around dementia that prevents open discussion, the misunderstanding that memory problems are part of normal ageing and the false belief that nothing can be done for those with dementia given that there is no cure.

Gill's Narrative 2.4: It's dementia

'I am still replaying that doctor's appointment in my mind.

"Do you know what the problem is then, Doctor?"

"We may still need to run more tests to confirm our diagnosis but we think that Peter might have vascular dementia."

I remember Peter's gasp at this news. I mean, I was shocked as well. The word "dementia" resounding in my head, my mind full of fearful images and connotations. I could only picture very frail and elderly figures sitting placidly and staring into space. I felt absolutely numb and remember reaching out and grasping Peter's hand tightly.

Isn't dementia an old person's illness? Peter is only 57. I know his memory is not as good as in the past but that can be explained by many things. Look at the new lease of life being enjoyed by his ex-colleague who took early retirement.

"I'm sorry, Mr and Mrs Lawrence, but the assessments we have carried out, particularly the brain scan, indicate a shrinkage of brain tissue and would confirm this diagnosis."'

- *At this 'turning point' for the Lawrence family, what constructive comment or advice could you offer Gill and Peter?*

Gill's narrative shows the impact and resonance caused by a single word, 'dementia'. They found it difficult to comprehend in part due to the connotations of this condition relating to old age, helplessness and incapacitated individuals, not fitting someone as young and seemingly robust as Peter. In this instance the diagnosis confirms vascular dementia. The process up to this date has evidently primed them to expect further tests and perhaps changes and refinements to the diagnosis given here. Gill's feelings about this continuation of testing are clearly expressed showing despair and extreme irritation. The diagnosis was given to Gill and Peter together and delivered verbally. The words 'we think it might be...' illustrates the areas of inconclusiveness that still exist, coupled with the phrase 'we may still need to run more tests'. Whilst this is totally understandable it can also signify something of the uncertainty and hesitation held by practitioners in such instances. In Mastwyk *et al.*'s (2014) study, most respondents (involving the person being tested and family carers) thought that a direct approach was best when presenting a dementia diagnosis, and that both written information and compassion demonstrated by the doctor and an opportunity to ask questions would be helpful. They want the support of a family member or friend when they are told of their diagnosis and they would like a written summary to refer to afterwards.

It is unquestionably a life-altering moment for the individual and significant others, heralding the start of a journey into what is largely the unknown. Birt *et al.* (2017) posit that disclosing a dementia diagnosis to those outside the family can help people move out of the liminal state and along a journey towards living well with dementia. The decision to disclose a diagnosis may be actively managed by the person as a way of retaining previous status and so potentially protecting the former self. Telling others of their dementia diagnosis creates opportunities to take control of social situations and use strategies to reduce the risk of stigma or embarrassment.

Young Dementia UK provides facts and figures on the common types of dementia in young people. Highlighting the difficulties of diagnosing people who are at working age, the statistics cited are likely to be inaccurate and may not reflect the true number of people, given many people's reluctance to seek help or the GP's attributing of symptoms to stress or depression.

Types of dementia in younger people (Young Dementia UK 2019)

- Alzheimer's disease – 33 per cent of young people with dementia. It is the most common form of dementia.
- Vascular dementia – 20 per cent of young people with dementia. It is the second most common form of dementia.
- Fronto-temporal dementia – 12 per cent of young people with dementia, commonly occurring between the ages of 45 to 65. There is evidence of family history in 40 per cent of people diagnosed.
- Korsakoff's syndrome – 10 per cent of young people with dementia, most commonly associated with alcohol abuse. Caused by a lack of vitamin B1 (thiamine).
- Dementia with Lewy bodies – 10 per cent of young people with dementia.
- Around 15 per cent of young people with dementia have conditions

that can lead to dementia and these include Parkinson's disease, Huntington's disease and Creutzfeldt-Jakob disease.

The interpersonal process of discussing a diagnosis requires attention to how information is conveyed. In a practical sense this could entail who is told, what and how they are told and the impact of this disclosure (Carpenter and Dave 2004). At this time thoughts may gravitate around differing expectations and life changes and may be spoken or not by the person with their diagnosis and family members. Karnieli-Miller *et al.* (2012) found family companions having more clear-cut expectations around the diagnostic process. In terms of dissatisfaction, companions complained about a lack of information or of tailored follow-up processes for implementing recommendations provided by the clinic. Patients' concerns stemmed mostly from how information was communicated and the outcome.

ACTIVITY 2.7

Previously, you were asked what would be the 'best' time for a dementia diagnosis to be given. Now consider the interpersonal process of 'diagnosis disclosure'.

If in a practitioner role, what information could I offer?

If in a familial role, what information would I want?

Are there any differences between your two responses?

Differences and discrepancies have historically existed between practitioners and carers. Connell *et al.* (2004) found caregivers recounting a highly negative emotional response to the disclosure, whereas many physicians reported that families had handled the information well. Caregivers expressed a range of preferences for how the diagnosis should have been disclosed ranging from a direct approach to having the physician ease them more steadily into the results. The need for improved doctor–patient communication and increased attention to caregiver needs was one of the main recommendations from Grossberg *et al.*'s (2010) study.

There are certain dilemmas experienced by practitioners around the disclosure process. Laakkonen *et al.* (2008) studied the experiences of spousal caregivers relating to the receipt of a dementia diagnosis and subsequent care received. Ninety-three per cent of caregivers reported that the dementia diagnosis had been disclosed openly to their spouse. Ninety-seven per cent preferred that physicians openly inform patients of the dementia diagnosis, although 55 per cent of their spouses with Alzheimer's disease had developed depressive symptoms after the disclosure. The responses in this qualitative study indicated that many caregivers felt grief and anxiety around the diagnosis disclosure. They also expressed feelings of loneliness and uncertainty about how to deal with follow-up care for dementia. A question commonly considered concerns whether or not it is anticipated that individuals really want to know (or not) about their diagnosis. Mormont *et al.* (2012) found that although the disclosure of the diagnosis of Alzheimer's disease is recommended by several guidelines, many clinicians are not announcing the diagnosis to their patients. One of the main arguments against disclosure is the fear of a depressive reaction. In their study:

- Twenty-nine per cent of participants said they suffered when the diagnosis was disclosed and 5 per cent wished they had not been informed.
- Four per cent felt more sad or depressed.
- Fourteen per cent felt more anxious since the disclosure.
- In 85 per cent of cases, the caregivers thought that the disclosure was useful. If they could go back in time and decide whether to disclose the diagnosis or not, only 4 per cent of caregivers would retrospectively disagree to disclose the diagnosis to the patient.

Robinson *et al.*'s (2011) research concluded that the vast majority of people with dementia wished to know their diagnosis. The key challenges for the person with dementia were regarded as coming to terms with losses on multiple levels. Although there may be short-term distress, the majority of people with dementia do not appear to experience long-term negative effects on their psychological health. For family carers, becoming the main decision-maker and adjusting to increased responsibility were common concerns. Interestingly, they found the term 'Alzheimer's disease' having more negative connotations than the broader term 'dementia'.

Lin *et al.* (2005) found reasons for favouring disclosure including a patient's or family member's right to know, the possibility of assistance in coping with and understanding dementia, and slowing down the progression of the disease with early treatment. They further asserted reasons for favouring the withholding of disclosure including the risk of causing the patient emotional disturbance, worsening the disease, the irrelevance of disclosure to drug therapy and the possibility of causing suicidal ideation. According to Holroyd, Turnbull and Wolf (2002), family members were significantly more likely to have been told the diagnosis and symptoms to expect in dementia than the patients themselves. Half of the families involved felt they were not given enough information regarding dementia. This decision can extend further with carers in favour of withholding information from patients as found in Shimizu *et al.*'s (2008) research. Both clinicians and patients experience avoidance in relation to the diagnosis, which includes the process of denial (Milby *et al.* 2017).

From a cultural perspective, Tuerk and Sauer (2015) reported on the findings of a small London-based study and the findings that people from African-Caribbean backgrounds are on average eight years younger when diagnosed with dementia compared with the white population and have lower scores on cognitive testing, indicating more advanced disease at presentation. Vascular dementia is thought to be the most common form of dementia among minority ethnic communities in the UK (particularly South Asian and black Caribbean), affecting 22 per cent of those living with dementia. This is due to the higher prevalence of risk factors such as diabetes, hypertension and cardiovascular disease (Moriarty *et al.* 2011). Young-onset dementia (affecting those under the age of 65 years) has also been found to be more common among minority ethnic groups, accounting for 6 per cent of the population living with dementia compared to 2 per cent of the white British population with dementia (Knapp *et al.* 2007).

As Vernooij-Dassen *et al.* (2006) assert, whilst the disclosure of dementia occurs at a single point in time, its impact should be seen as a process. Interviews revealed a gradual process of realization amongst participants of what the diagnosis meant, resulting in important subtle changes in understandings of dementia and personal relationships. The shock caused by a dementia diagnosis can be related to expectations and perceived connotations. Helga Rohra (2016, p.45), diagnosed with dementia with Lewy bodies at the age of 54, reflects upon the stereotypical image we have:

> People with dementia are old, in need of care, helpless and dependent. They can't look after themselves or their children, and certainly can't live unsupervised in their own home. They need care, if possible round the clock, because they are always running away, getting lost, are inappropriately dressed and have simply 'lost it'.

Prior to her diagnosis she worked as a translator and was now facing a very uncertain and pessimistic future with her independence threatened:

> The end is nigh... I have no idea how I got from the consulting room back into the waiting room. I was sobbing and there was no one to come to my aid... Somehow or other I got out into the street. I felt so wretched, so dizzy. Incapable about thinking about the next step. (Rohra 2016, p.43)

Christine Bryden (2018) was bluntly informed that she had probable dementia and should retire from work immediately and that she should not be in any position of responsibility. This is echoed by Kate Swaffer's (2016) narrative illustrative of what she refers to as a process of Prescribed Disengagement®. What emerges powerfully here is the sense of shock in some instances fuelled by the lack of sensitivity or fairly hopeless anticipated progression communicated by their diagnosing practitioners. These issues will be examined more in the following chapter as we continue to follow the Lawrence family's dementia journey.

How true could this be today?

The theme of 'How true could this be today?' asks you to consider reframing an observation from the past. This commentary had an influence in informing thinking at that time whilst also determining opinions of the day. A number of questions will encourage you to consider its relevance in the here and now, such as: have national opinions changed or not? Do you agree or not with these comments? What has influenced your attitudes?

Background information: Talcott Parsons (1951) offered a commentary on what could happen as a consequence of a diagnosis, with the origins of the phrase 'sick role' being traced back to his work. A view was expressed that a diagnosis may provide an explanation for symptoms, lead to decisions regarding treatment, offer a prognosis and create certain expectations...where the sick are seen as failing in some way to fulfil their role(s) within society.

- What are your views on this observation from the 1950s?
- Do you believe it still exists or not?
- What personal and/or professional evidence have you for your comments?

Concluding thoughts

This chapter began by inviting you to accompany Gill, Peter and their family on their journey through the maze of tests and assessments, through to the eventual receipt of a dementia diagnosis. As an acquaintance of the family you have been able to access regular updates courtesy of Gill's narratives as to what was being experienced. This privileged perspective facilitates appreciation of the lived internal experience and greater understanding of what the family's support needs might be. Hopefully you have been able to get a sense of the feelings involved and better understand why rationalizations and compensatory strategies can be employed as a way of coping with the uncertainty around Peter's behaviours. Engagement with this process may have evoked in you similar feelings to those of the Lawrence family and an encouragement to explore what you feel and think about the diagnostic process. As one could imagine, after leaving the practitioner's office the reality of what individuals have been told will start to sink in, leaving people with much to process. The next part of the Lawrence family's journey covers the growing reality and appreciation of the diagnosis as they seek to make sense of this change in their lives.

PERSONAL LEARNING

What was your past knowledge and understanding, what new learning have you achieved and how could this inform your future personal and/or professional interventions?

As a 'family member', my new learning includes ....

....

On reading the first-person narratives, my new learning includes

....

INTERVENTIONS

Be mindful that whatever comments are offered should be realistic, achievable and person-centred. Also that the feelings conveyed and observations made reinforce that 'tests are being conducted and a diagnosis is imminent' for the individual and significant other people in their life.

The types of interventions could include ....

....

References

Ahmad, S., Orrell, M., Iliffe, S. and Gracie, A. (2010). 'GPs' attitudes, awareness, and practice regarding early diagnosis of dementia.' *British Journal of General Practice 60* (578), 360–365.

Alzheimer's Association (2019). *Visiting your Doctor.* Accessed on 11/10/19 at www.alz.org/alzheimers-dementia/diagnosis/visiting-your-doctor.

Alzheimer's Society (2019a). *Concerned about Someone Else's Memory Problems?* Accessed on 11/10/19 at www.alzheimers.org.uk/about-dementia/symptoms-and-diagnosis/how-dementia-progresses/concerned-about-someone-elses-memory-problems.

Alzheimer's Society (2019b). *Beginning Again: A Message of Hope.* Accessed on 11/10/19 at www.alzheimers.org.uk/dementia-together-magazine/apr-may-2019/beginning-again-message-hope.

Alzheimer's Society Canada (2018). *Preparing for your Doctor's Visit.* Accessed 5/11/19 at https://alzheimer.ca/en/Home/About-dementia/Diagnosis/Preparing-for-your-doctor-s-visit.

Bastos, C. (2012). 'Educational level in the diagnostic of dementias: a research with elderly patients.' *European Psychiatry 27* (Supplement 1), 1.

BBC (2006). *One Life: My Life on a Post It Note.* Accessed on 7/9/17 at https://forum.alzheimers.org.uk/threads/bbc-one-life-my-life-on-a-post-it-note.3357.

Beaumont, H. (2009). *Losing Clive to Younger Onset Dementia.* London: Jessica Kingsley Publishers.

Birt, L., Poland, F. Csipke, E. and Charlesworth, G. (2017). 'Shifting dementia discourses from deficit to active citizenship.' *Sociology of Health and Illness. 39* (2), 199–211.

Bond, J., Stave, C., Sganga, A., Vincenzino, O., O'Connell, B. and Stanley, R.L. (2005). 'Inequalities in dementia care across Europe: key findings of the Facing Dementia Survey.' *International Journal of Clinical Practice 59*, 8–14.

Brodaty, H., Pond, D. and Kemp, N. (2002). 'The GPCOG: a new screening test for dementia designed for general practice.' *Journal of American Geriatric Society 50* (3), 530–534.

Brooke, P and Bullock, R. (1999). 'Validation of a 6 item cognitive impairment test with a view to primary care use.' *International Journal of Geriatric Psychiatry 14* (11), 936–940.

Brown, J. and Hillam, J. (2004). *Dementia: Your Questions Answered.* China: Churchill Livingstone.

Bryden, C. (2018). *Will I Still Be Me? Finding a Continuing Sense of Self in the Lived Experience of Dementia.* London: Jessica Kingsley Publishers.

Burns, A. (2012). 'Primary Care Holds the Key to Raising Quality of Dementia Patients' Lives.' *Guardian Professional.* 24 September.

Bryden, C. (2005). *Dancing with Dementia.* London: Jessica Kingsley Publishers.

Campbell, S., Manthorpe, J., Samsi, K., Abley, C., Robinson, L., Watts, S., Bond, J. and Keady, J. (2016). 'Living with uncertainty: mapping the transition from pre-diagnosis to a diagnosis of dementia.' *Journal of Aging Studies 37*, 40–47.

Carling, C. (2012). *But Then Something Happened.* Cambridge: Golden Books.

Carpenter, B. and Dave, J. (2004). 'Disclosing a dementia diagnosis: a review of opinion and practice, and a proposed research agenda.' *Gerontologist 44* (2), 149–158.

Connell, C.M., Boise, L., Stuckey, J.C., Holmes, S.B. and Hudson, M.L. (2004). 'Attitudes toward the diagnosis and disclosure of dementia among family caregivers and primary care physicians.' *Gerontologist 44* (4), 500–507.

Davis, R. (1989). *My Journey into Alzheimer's Disease.* Illinois: Tyndale House.

Dementia Australia (2019). *Frequently asked Questions.* Accessed on 10/11/19 at www.dementia.org.au.

Department of Health and Social Care (2009). *Living Well with Dementia: A New National Dementia Strategy.* London: Department of Health and Social Care.

Dhedhi, S.A., Swinglehurst, D. and Russell, J. (2014). 'Timely diagnosis of dementia: what does it mean? A narrative analysis of GPs' accounts.' *BMJ Open 4* (3), 1–9.

Dillon, K. (2016). 'Adult children who are caregivers of parents diagnosed with dementia: the relationship between anticipatory grief, depression, and closeness to the parent prior to the diagnosis.' *Dissertation Abstracts International: Section B: The Sciences and Engineering.* Vol.76 (9-B(E)).

Folstein, M., Folstein, S. and McHugh, P. (1975). 'Mini-Mental State: a practical method for grading the cognitive state of patients for the clinician.' *Journal of Psychiatric Research 12*, 189–198.

Gainotti, G. and Marra, C. (1994). 'Some aspects of memory disorders clearly distinguish dementia of the Alzheimer's type from depressive pseudo-dementia.' *Journal of Clinical and Experimental Neuropsychology 16* (1), 65–78.

Gofton, T. and Weaver, D.F. (2006). 'Challenges in the clinical diagnosis of Alzheimer's disease: influence of "family coaching" on the Mini-Mental State Examination.' *American Journal of Alzheimer's Disease and other Dementias 21* (2), 109–112.

Grossberg, G.T., Christensen, D.D., Griffith, P.A., Kerwin, D.R., Hunt, G. and Hall, E.J. (2010). 'The art of sharing the diagnosis and management of Alzheimer's disease with patients and caregivers: recommendations of an expert consensus panel.' *Primary Care Companion to the Journal of Clinical Psychiatry 12* (1), e1–e9.

Healthtalk (n.d.). *Interview 31*. Accessed on 12/1/18 at www.healthtalk.org/carers-people-dementia/interview-31.

Holroyd, S., Turnbull, Q. and Wolf, A. (2002). 'What are patients and their families told about the diagnosis of dementia? Results of a family survey.' *International Journal of Geriatric Psychiatry 17* (3), 218–221.

Houchen, A. (2010). 'Strained to the Limit.' In L. Whitman (ed.) *Telling Tales About Dementia: Experiences of Caring*. London: Jessica Kingsley Publishers.

Husband, H. (1999). 'Psychological consequences of learning a diagnosis of dementia: three case examples.' *Aging and Mental Health 3* (2), 179–183.

Jamieson-Craig, R., Scior, K., Chan, T., Fenton, C. and Strydom, A. (2010). 'Reliance on carer reports of early symptoms of dementia among adults with intellectual disabilities.' *Journal of Policy and Practice in Intellectual Disabilities 7* (1), 34–41.

Karnieli-Miller, O., Werner, P., Aharon-Peretz, J., Sinoff, G. and Eidelman, S. (2012). 'Expectations, experiences, and tensions in the Memory Clinic: the process of diagnosis disclosure of dementia within a triad.' *International Psychogeriatrics 24* (11), 1756–1770.

Knapp, M., Prince, M. and Albanese, E. (2007). *Dementia UK. A Report to the Alzheimer's Society on the Prevalence and Economic Cost of Dementia in the UK.* London: King's College London and London School of Economics.

Laakkonen, M., Raivio, M., Eloniemi-Sulkava, U., Saarenheimo, M., Pietila, M., Tilvis, R. and Pitkala, K. (2008). 'How do elderly spouse care givers of people with Alzheimer disease experience the disclosure of dementia diagnosis and subsequent care?' *Journal of Medical Ethics 34* (6), 427–430.

Lian, Y., Xiao, L., Zeng, F., Wu, X., Wang, Z. and Ren, H. (2017). 'The experiences of people with dementia and their caregivers in dementia diagnosis.' *Journal of Alzheimer's Disease 59* (4), 1203–1211.

Lin, K., Liao, Y., Wang, P. and Liu, H. (2005). 'Family members favor disclosing the diagnosis of Alzheimer's disease.' *International Psychogeriatrics 17* (4), 679–688.

Marzanski, M. (2000). 'On telling the truth to patients with dementia.' *Western Journal of Medicine 173* (5), 318–323.

Mastwyk, M., Ames, D., Ellis, K., Chiu, E. and Dow, B. (2014). 'Disclosing a dementia diagnosis: what do patients and family consider important?' *International Psychogeriatrics 26* (8), 1263–1272.

Milby, E., Murphy, G. and Winthrop, A. (2017). 'Diagnosis disclosure in dementia: understanding the experiences of clinicians and patients who have recently given or received a diagnosis.' *The International Journal of Social Research and Practice 16* (5), 611–628.

Moriarty, J., Sharif, N. and Robinson, J. (2011). *Black and Minority Ethnic People with Dementia and Their Access to Support and Services.* London: Social Care Institute for Excellence.

Mormont, E., de Fays, K. and Jamart, J. (2012). 'Experiences of the patients and their caregivers regarding the disclosure of the diagnosis of Alzheimer's disease: a Belgian retrospective survey.' *Acta Neurologica Belgica 112* (3), 249–254.

Nasreddine, Z., Phillips, N. and Bedrian, V. (2005). 'The Montreal Cognitive Assessment (MoCA): a brief screening tool for mild cognitive impairment.' *Journal of American Geriatric Society 53* (4), 695–699.

National Institute for Health and Care Excellence (2018). *Dementia: Assessment, Management and Support for People Living with Dementia and their Carers*. Accessed on 18/06/20 at https://www.nice.org.uk/guidance/ng97.

NHS (2017). *Tests for Diagnosing Dementia.* Accessed on 31/10/17 at www.nhs.uk/conditions/dementia/diagnosis-tests.

Oliver, K. (2019). *Dear Alzheimer's: A Diary of Living with Dementia.* London: Jessica Kingsley Publishers.

Parsons, T. (1951). *The Social System.* Glencoe: The Free Press.

Perry-Young, L., Owen, G., Kelly, S. and Owens, C. (2018). 'How people come to recognise a problem and seek medical help for a person showing early signs of dementia: a systematic review and meta-ethnography.' *Dementia 17* (1), 34–60.

Pratt, R. (2002). 'Nobody's Ever Asked Me how I Felt.' In H. Wilkinson (ed.) *The Perspectives of People with Dementia: Research Methods and Motivation*. London: Jessica Kingsley Publishers.

Pratt, R. and Wilkinson, H. (2001). *'Tell Me the Truth': The Effect of Being Told the Diagnosis of Dementia from the Perspective of the Person with Dementia*. London: Mental Health Foundation.

Pratt, R. and Wilkinson, H. (2003). 'A psychosocial model of understanding the experience of receiving a diagnosis of dementia.' *The International Journal of Social Research and Practice 2* (2), 181–199.

Qureshi, K. and Hodkinson, H. (1974). 'Evaluation of a Ten-Question Mental State in the institutionalised elderly.' *Age and Ageing 3*, 152–157.

Robinson, L., Gemski, A., Abley, C., Bond, J., Keady, J., Campbell, S., Samsi, K. and Manthorpe, J. (2011). 'The transition to dementia: individual and family experiences of receiving a diagnosis: a review.' *International Psychogeriatrics 23* (7), 1026–1043.

Robinson, L., Tang, E. and Taylor, J. (2015). *Dementia: Timely Diagnosis and Early Intervention*. Accessed on 15/11/16 at www.bmj.com/content/350/bmj.h3029.

Roe, C., Xiong, C., Miller, P. and Morris, J. (2007). 'Education and Alzheimer's disease without the dementia: support for the cognitive reserve hypothesis.' *Neurology 68* (3), 223–228.

Rohra, H. (2016). *Dementia Activist*. London: Jessica Kingsley Publishers.

Ross, A. (2009). An assessment of anticipatory grief as experienced by family caregivers of individuals with dementia. *Dissertation Abstracts International: Section B: The Sciences and Engineering*. 69(10-B), 6433.

Samsi, K., Abley, C., Campbell, S., Keady, J., Manthorpe, J., Robinson, L., Watts, S. and Bond, J. (2014). 'Negotiating a labyrinth: experiences of assessment and diagnostic journey in cognitive impairment and dementia.' *International Journal of Geriatric Psychiatry 29* (1), 58–67.

Shimizu, M., Raicher, I., Takahashi, D., Caramelli, P. and Nitrini, R. (2008). 'Disclosure of the diagnosis of Alzheimer's disease: caregivers' opinions in a Brazilian sample.' *Arquivos de Neuro-Psiquiatria 66* (3-B), 625–630.

Shulman, K., Shedletsky, R. and Silver, I. (1986). 'The challenge of time: clock drawing and cognitive functioning in the elderly.' *International Journal of Geriatric Psychiatry 1*, 135–140.

Swaffer, K. (2016). *What the Hell Happened to My Brain? Living Beyond Dementia*. London: Jessica Kingsley Publishers.

Teel, C. and Carson, P. (2005). 'Family experiences in the journey through dementia diagnosis and care.' *Journal of Family Nursing 9* (1), 38–58.

Tuerk, R. and Sauer, J. (2015). 'Dementia in a black and minority ethnic population: characteristics of presentation to an inner London memory service.' *British Journal of Psychiatry Bulletin 39* (4), 162–166.

UCL Department of Mental Health Services (2005). *Choice Fact Sheets*. Accessed on 19/3/15 at www.bmj.com/content/suppl/2010/08/18/bmj.c4184.DC1/livg719658.ww1_default.pdf.

Vernooij-Dassen, M., Derksen, E., Scheltens, P. and Moniz-Cook, E. (2006). 'Receiving a diagnosis of dementia: the experience over time.' *The International Journal of Social Research and Practice 5* (3), 397–410.

Whalley, L. and Breitner, J. (2002). *Fast Facts: Dementia*. Washington: Health Press International.

Wilkinson, H. and Milne, A. (2003). 'Sharing a diagnosis of dementia – learning from the patient perspective.' *Aging and Mental Health 7* (4), 300–307.

Young Dementia UK (2019). *Types of Dementia in Younger People*. Accessed on 8/9/19 at www.youngdementiauk.org/types-dementia-younger-people-0.

Part 2

Living with Dementia

Chapter 3

Making Sense of Things

Introduction

The main feature within this chapter explores the impact a diagnosis of dementia can have on the individual concerned and their family. In the immediate aftermath feelings of shock and bewilderment can give way to other conflicting emotions including denial, despair, anger, frustration, anxiety and sadness. A generic diagnosis does not explain how an individual receives this information as each member has their own unique comprehension and distinct feeling about what the term 'dementia' means to them. This word resonates strongly, fuelling fears and fantasies about the months and years ahead. It is not surprisingly a period where individuals relate feeling overwhelmed and struggling to make sense of what is taking place within their family group. There is also an evident need for learning in relation to what can help people cope with the months and years ahead. The myriad of feelings evoked will be experienced differently across the family with members having their own needs concerning emotional support. A further problem is the issue around who to tell and how much to reveal about a family member's diagnosis, given the fears and uncertainties about others' reactions. It is a time with families experiencing significant disruption to their lives, having a clear need for assistance in navigating the road that lies before them.

The story so far

Peter and Gill are currently struggling to come to terms with the news they have received. They have endured months of assessments, scans and tests in what was a very stressful and anxiety-provoking time and an agonizing wait for results. Family members had suspected that there was a serious problem for some time now with Peter's behaviour becoming harder to explain away. This had all placed a significant strain on relationships within the family. Hearing the word 'dementia' spoken by the doctor came as a complete shock. Peter's initial response was 'How can that be? It's an old person's condition and I'm only 57.'

Chapter themes

Stokes, Combes and Stokes' (2014) research identified four main themes emerging for individuals with dementia and their partners following their receipt of diagnosis. They included an insufficiency of information; low levels of societal understanding and associated stigma; difficulties with adjustment; and the need for greater partnership working.

This highlights a number of significant factors, especially the need to understand what is happening and what this means for families and their lives ahead. Information will also be needed to make sense of what has occurred and the potential causes. The need to make adjustments points towards a need for emotional support, helping to cope with the shock that will undoubtedly be felt. Tackling stigma and engaging partnership working starts with talking and engaging with others.

The themes in this chapter will include:

- Emotional support needs – 'We are in shock'
- Implications – 'What happens to us now?'
- Initial follow-up support – 'We are in need of information'
- Making sense – 'Why me? Why us?'
- Telling others – 'Who should we tell? What can we say?'

Emotional support needs ('We are in shock')

The receipt of a dementia diagnosis will be startling and require time to work through. Ken H (Young Dementia UK 2019) was diagnosed with Alzheimer's disease in his mid-fifties and recalls:

> Being diagnosed with dementia is brutal. It is horrendous. Only someone who has been through it can understand. You are given a mental death sentence. I felt the doctor left me in that frame of mind and left me to pick up the pieces of my life. Someone needs to give you hope, and tell you that you won't be a burden. You have to realise that this is not the end. You walk away and nothing's changed but everything is different.

This narrative illustrates a person in deep shock focusing predominantly upon the negative impact that it is anticipated this condition will have upon their life. Phrases such as 'pick up the pieces of my life', 'mental death sentence' and 'someone needs to give you hope' illustrate very keenly a sense of desperation and hopelessness. This section examines such feelings and what individuals' support needs are through this difficult and emotion-laden transition. There is a need to make adjustments for the near future and longer term with significant emotional support required to cope with the outcome of this diagnosis.

Gill's Narrative 3.1: In a daze

'I still can't get my head around what has happened to us and just feel utterly bewildered. How can Peter have dementia at his age? I can't concentrate or properly apply myself to anything and am not sleeping well at present. The house looks an absolute tip. Peter is also struggling to make sense of the news and just seems to be in a constant daze. We have both worked hard all our lives, bringing up a family and should by rights now be expecting to enjoy some welcome time together, not having this blasted curse to contend with. It is just so unfair!

I am already struggling with the florist shop and will have to somehow divide my time even more. We should also be paying more attention to Tom who is now in high school. The future was once pretty much about watching the kids grow up and then me and Peter enjoying some time together. We always wanted to travel and see a bit of the world. What now? Do I have to helplessly watch Peter deteriorate, unable to do anything about it? It is far too soon. Tom has friends with grandparents who have dementia. How will he make sense of this being his father?'

- *If you were Ashleigh, what could you initially say:*
    - *to Mum when she was informed about Dad's diagnosis?*
    - *to Matt who is now living away about Mum and Dad's diagnosis news?*
    - *to Tom who is still living at home?*

Gill's narrative illustrates her sense of bewilderment and struggle to accommodate the news that she and Peter have received. There is a strong sense of injustice and unfairness related in connection to the potential loss of their future plans and projected time together. Life is now seen as being very uncertain and muddled with the house 'an absolute tip' symbolizing the chaos and devastation that has visited their lives. Essentially, this is a family in shock and in desperate need of emotional support and guidance to help prepare them for the changes lying ahead of them. A diagnosis of young-onset dementia may have marked consequences for the person, and these can include having to take early retirement, experiencing financial pressures and negotiating the psychological challenges of coming to terms with cognitive decline (Draper and Withall 2016).

ACTIVITY 3.1

In the introductory chapter we asked you to express your thoughts and feelings about the term 'diagnosis of dementia'. Returning to your original responses, ask yourself the following:

Why do I hold these beliefs?

When and where did my attitudes become established?

How receptive would I be to changing my attitudes?

Being in receipt of a diagnosis of young-onset dementia presents many particular challenges for the individual and significant other people in their life. Innes, Szymczynska and Stark (2014) highlight the importance of post-diagnostic support and state that without it, government targets for diagnosis are simply quota targets, rather than what they should be: the means to improve service experiences. We can review this against the drive for earlier dementia diagnosis (Department of Health 2009), which is measured by De Vugt and Verhey (2013) against the level of support offered. They acknowledge the drawbacks of an early diagnosis outweighing the benefits where people are left with little support. Gill's narrative above illustrates the sense of shock and disbelief felt with both Peter and Gill struggling to comprehend what has occurred. They share a clear sense of uncertainty over what the implications are for them in the present and future, both temporal states that have suddenly become daunting and unclear. The multitude of emotions evoked will need time and support to acknowledge and begin to work through. If we look at what is routinely offered, this includes counselling and follow-up help and advice. Frenette and Beauchemin (2005) recommend that family physicians offer anticipatory counselling to those recently diagnosed with dementia as well as directing caregivers towards resources for psychological support. There is a key need for this especially given the findings in Zubatsky's (2015) study with participants revealing a lack of awareness concerning available community resources and with none accessed during the initial stage of a family member's diagnosis. Contributory issues included the experiencing of depression as well as feeling that concerns were unacknowledged by healthcare providers.

Figure 3.1 shows in a diagram some of the 'diagnostic dynamics' for the person with dementia, their family and friends. You may wish to expand upon this and add your own thoughts.

Personal dynamics – concerns about the well-being of the person diagnosed/quality of life and role transition/lifestyle changes/loss/uncertainty and reliance on others/cultural concerns/treatments/stigma or not/...

Increased numbers of people being diagnosed

Societal dynamics – commercial concerns and adequate services/burdens and perceptions of dementia/health and social care services/cultural concerns/treatments/stigma or not/...

Figure 3.1 Diagnostic dynamics

The space and 'permission' to address feelings evoked is vital and necessary. The late author Terry Pratchett, who was himself diagnosed with dementia, advocated the need for people to acknowledge and name the emotions involved, helping to normalize and validate their experience. This engages a sense of *permission-giving*, for individuals to own their feelings as well as seeking a means of self-expression. What is felt is something that is unique to each person and their individual characteristics and personal support mechanisms. The need for space and guidance to process one's experience is vividly outlined within Keith Oliver's (2019, p.63) narrative. Initially prescribed antidepressant medication in response he reflected: 'I'm not depressed. I'm frustrated, I'm bored. I'm unstimulated, I'm intellectually drifting, but, certainly, I'm not depressed. I need a challenge. I need a focus. I don't need a drug.'

This is a telling statement and challenges practitioners to actively listen to what those newly diagnosed with dementia might be telling us or asking for.

The Alzheimer's Society provide a range of factsheets and booklets to support individuals through this process, which includes their 'Understanding Your Diagnosis' publications, as related to specific types of dementia (Alzheimer's, vascular dementia, dementia with Lewy bodies, fronto-temporal dementia, young-onset dementia). A section within each of these is titled 'Coping with your feelings' and acknowledges commonly experienced emotions such as shock, disbelief, denial, fear, guilt and loss. The booklet specifically aimed at those with young-onset dementia attempts to connect directly with those affected with phrases such as 'you are not alone' and 'there is no "right" or "wrong" way to feel' (Alzheimer's Society 2017). The acknowledgement and validation of likely feelings continues with suggestions for coping and managing feelings and recognizing that 'Many people feel frustrated or angry, have a sense that it isn't fair, or ask "why me?", "why now?"'

This reflects Gill's feelings of injustice, something commonly felt by others diagnosed with young-onset dementia. Christine Bryden (2018, p.21) was told by her specialist that she would likely be in full-time care within a few years and it would be only a few years more before she died. Not surprisingly this competent and very able woman, diagnosed at the age of 46, felt paralysed with fear for her future: 'Hanging over me were the rolling and ominous black clouds of the loss of self that were supposed to occur with dementia. Would I know my daughters? Would I even know myself? Who would I be when I died?'

In Aminzadeh *et al.*'s (2007) study examining the emotional impact of diagnosis disclosure on those recently diagnosed with dementia, responses included grief related to actual or anticipated losses. As Gill's narrative highlights, this can include all of the experiences and planned activities that families would now not be able to enjoy in the years ahead and includes the many plans and expectations for their retirement. The extent of the anticipated losses is especially felt at younger ages with the perception of larger spans of time and a wider range of experiences impacted upon. The sense of shock and bewilderment is starkly illustrated by Yvonne Hague's narrative with her expression of the struggle to come to terms with her husband's diagnosis of dementia at the extremely young age of 40 (Morris and Morris 2010). She writes of her determination to remain positive for both her ten-year-old daughter and her husband. Similarly, Daniel Bradbury, married and with two-year-old twins, was diagnosed with dementia at the age of 30. He featured in BBC 1's documentary *Our Dementia Choir* (2019) speaking expressively about daily challenges and his fears for his family's future. When reviewing experiences such as these, the impact upon a family's daily life is powerfully felt. This can be in response to their day-to-day functioning, enforced changes in roles and impending loss. It is important to note though that such an impact need not be lessened if those diagnosed are in their seventies or eighties.

Prince *et al.* (2015) have identified the impact of dementia on three interrelated levels:

- individual with dementia (impaired quality of life and reduced life expectancy)
- family and friends (witnessing the deterioration in the health of their loved one)
- wider society (cost of providing health and social care and cost of lost productivity).

At this stage it will be hard for individuals to know who to turn to for support. Agencies such as the Oxfordshire-based Young Dementia UK provide practical and emotional support for partners, children and parents to adapt to living with a person with young-onset dementia. They signpost potential feelings of desperation: 'Do not be surprised if you find yourself wanting to shout about the injustice of what is happening or cannot stop crying.'

This agency also urges those affected to ask for help, talk to people about what they are experiencing and to allow themselves space to work through difficulties. Given the considerable span of time that on average elapses before a diagnosis has been confirmed we can only guess at the strain that family members have been through coping largely in isolation.

EXERCISE: WHAT IF IT'S NOT ALZHEIMER'S DISEASE?

This exercise asks the reader to consider their 'felt experiences' and understanding of the ways vascular dementia is researched, causative lifestyles and narratives. (See Chapter 8.)

Implications ('What happens to us now?')

The previous section explored the initial feelings of shock experienced by families given a dementia diagnosis. Following this a period of time will be needed for individuals to begin taking stock of what this means for them and their future lives. As can be imagined the perceived implications are likely to be focused strongly around restrictions in connection with relationships, activities, employment and social life. As Jackson (2010, p.54) recalls:

> When the formal diagnosis of vascular dementia was made, my feelings were of devastation and catastrophe. I was overcome with a great fear of the future, as well as deep sorrow and sympathy for my husband in what seemed a kind of death sentence.

This narrative shows the extent of the perceived impact a diagnosis of dementia can bring with striking terms such as 'devastation' and 'catastrophe' stressed. It is understandable that in this initial stage attention is likely to be keenly focused upon projected losses and detrimental changes. This and wider issues are explored within this section.

Gill's Narrative 3.2: What does it mean?

'I am trying to get my head around what this diagnosis means for our family. What tensions are likely to emerge between us and will we still be able to cope? Peter seems crushed by the realization of his dementia and is drinking noticeably more. One of the hardest things for him I know is the contemplation of being a person with a "condition". Because it is "dementia" it makes acceptance much harder. He did remind me of a statement he made some years ago after visiting a great aunt with Alzheimer's saying "If I ever get dementia just shoot me."

What will happen with his work and what about my business? Matt is in his final year at university and finding it hard meeting all his expenses. I don't know how much we can continue helping him financially. How will Ashleigh and Tom take this news? It all seems so bleak and uncertain.'

- *What advice could you offer regarding:*
  - *Gill's present concerns about Peter?*
  - *Gill's well-being?*

Gill's narrative attempts to make sense of how the family will be impacted upon as well as the implications for her relationship with Peter. Her account has a predominantly pessimistic tone including the necessity for Peter to give up work and restrictions for her own working life with their associated financial impact. For Gill and the family, Peter's relatively young age will make acceptance of his condition all the more difficult. This is especially so if reflected against the stereotypical view of frail individuals sitting passively in nursing homes. Indeed, prevailing emotions amongst individuals recently diagnosed are noted as fear and anticipated shame, including socially stigmatizing images of 'vegetating elders' in care facilities (Moniz-Cook *et al.* 2006).

Participants in Clemerson, Walsh and Isaac's (2014) study, diagnosed with young-onset dementia, spoke of the shock and disbelief at their diagnosis particularly with the feeling of being too young to have this condition. This is reiterated by Harris (2004, p.17) who relates: 'Dementia is socially defined as an old person's disease. And although the definition of dementia has changed over time its correlation with the ageing process has not.'

To understand more about age distinctions it is worth considering the use of the term 'young-onset dementia', synonymous with 'early-onset dementia' and 'working-age dementia', and defined in the UK as anyone diagnosed with dementia under the age of 65 years. As noted previously there are over 42,000 younger people with dementia from a current incidence of 850,000 people in the UK. This is a substantial figure and indicates a prevalence rate higher than that assumed within societal perceptions.

What people endure following the delivery of a diagnosis is unique to them, although studies around the impact of a diagnosis of dementia on people aged under 65 years and their families reveal negative outcomes for both the individual and carers (Svanberg, Spector and Stott 2011). This is supported through numerous personal narratives with the initial impact upon receiving a diagnosis of dementia coming as an enormous and devastating shock.

ACTIVITY 3.2

Consider what the negative implications could be when a person receives a diagnosis:

- Negative behaviours could include ....
- Negative attitudes could include ....

Your responses to Activity 3.2 may be generic or specific in interpretation although we would like to ask you to be mindful that how a person engages with their diagnosis is a very individual experience. This unique personal experience therefore may involve a plethora of emotions and Robinson (2010) outlines feelings such as sadness, helplessness and anger. This is reflected in Clare *et al.*'s (2002) study with findings indicating that 40 per cent of people recently diagnosed with dementia experience anxiety and 17 per cent experience depression. Indeed, of major concern is the recognition of an increased suicide risk in the three-month period following diagnosis (Draper *et al.* 2009). Help is clearly needed for the families affected and, interestingly, lower levels of anxiety were noted amongst those attending a memory clinic, underlining the importance of early support for those diagnosed and their families, especially given the feelings of terror concerning the future. Indeed, Fortinsky (2009) recommends counselling interventions, support groups and the formation of partnerships between professionals and service-users and carers.

In Connell *et al.*'s (2009) study, family members strongly endorsed the benefits of obtaining a dementia diagnosis, including getting information, finding out what is wrong with their relative, and prompting future planning. This was offset against barriers such as the perceived lack of a cure and the belief that little can be done for someone with Alzheimer's disease. Nurock (2010) relates her emotional turmoil and anger over her husband's diagnosis as well as being fearful about their future social and financial position. What she felt was missing for her and her husband at this stage was any sense of hope or proper concern for his emotional well-being, resulting in his becoming depressed and exacerbating the grieving process she was going through. The need for help, understanding and acknowledgement is facilitated by peer-led resources such as the Alzheimer's Society's Talking Point discussion forum. This provides an invaluable platform for sharing experiences and feelings with others (service-users, carers and family members) who are undergoing related experiences. The following posting is illustrative of many others reflecting initial distress and fears about a family member's diagnosis:

> I haven't been able to stop crying yet. I'm so upset and so angry about what has been taken away from not only me but my children. They are 1 and 2, and I know they won't have that relationship with nanny. I can't call on my mum when the baby won't stop crying or to babysit. I don't know how I will deal with this in the years ahead, I feel so lost. (Alzheimer's Society 2019a)

ACTIVITY 3.3

What emotions can you observe from this first-person narrative (Alzheimer's Society 2019a)?

What support and/or practical help would you think it is helpful to offer?

The replies to this particular posting demonstrate a high degree of acknowledgement and appreciation as to what they might be going through with emotions such as anger, tearfulness, frustration and helplessness shared. There was also a fair degree of advice imparted, stressing the need to discuss emotions and experiences and keeping one's network of family, friends and neighbours open. This Talking Point forum is a vibrant resource providing individuals with opportunities to share information and resources as well as to support each other. Within the sections available, the 'Support from other members' area has thousands of discussion threads arranged under a variety of headings such as:

- I have a partner with dementia.
- I care for a person with dementia.
- I am recently diagnosed with dementia.

The number of people posting queries or replying helpfully to others shows a high level of support evidenced, for example:

> I'm a new member to the forum, think this is an amazing site and the help you guys give to each other leaves me speechless. Was wondering if I could pick your brains and ask for any advice – could do with talking to someone in the same boat.

The person posting goes on to relate details regarding their father's recent dementia diagnosis and difficulties in commencing a caring role. The responses received are empathic and supportive.

Many people can only wonder what it might feel like for the person who has a dementia diagnosis as well as the impact that this has upon a person's family. It is a life-changing moment heralding potential restrictions and difficulties as outlined by Christine Bryden (2015a, p.40):

> The diagnosis has changed our lives forever. Our lives become limited by the stigma we face in the world around us. It's like we have a target painted on our foreheads shouting out 'dementing' for all the world to see. People become awkward in our presence, are unsure of our behaviour, and our world becomes circumscribed by the stigma of our illness.

Kate Swaffer (2016, p.318) outlines further the initially perceived implications describing her dementia diagnosis as having a: 'significant emotional, financial and social cost and impact on the person with dementia, their families, and society. It disempowers, devalues, demeans and lowers self-esteem and very negatively impacts wellbeing and quality of life.'

These two narratives outline very powerfully the life-limiting powers that this condition can have. Indeed, as mentioned above, Swaffer's (2016) process of Prescribed Disengagement® conjures up an extreme sense of pessimism and hopelessness.

Gill's narrative alludes to Peter's impending need to finish working as well as worries for her own business and the consequent implications including financial restrictions. Arguably, being employed is an important life activity that can be considered as far more than just a means to earn a wage. Work also provides a person with membership of a social group and the opportunity to contribute and feel valued. It helps define a person's identity, social roles and social status as well as leading to better health outcomes, promoting full participation in society and improving quality of life (Waddell and Burton 2006).

ACTIVITY 3.4

Briefly outline the benefits of employment for a person.

Briefly outline the burdens of unemployment for a person.

From your two responses:

- How might this impact on an employed person with a dementia diagnosis?
- How might this impact on an unemployed person with a dementia diagnosis?
- What could these burdens be if a person was in their mid-life, or younger?

Chaplin and Davidson (2016) explored the experience of people who were working when dementia developed and found that some believed they were treated poorly and felt abandoned at work. There was a noticeable sense of added scrutiny and a lack of consultation over decisions impacting upon employees. Indeed, Chris, who was diagnosed with vascular dementia at the age of 60, negotiated a phased return to work but felt wholly unsupported, something not helped by the sight of seeing his desk moved to the corner of the room. He ended up going through a disciplinary process for people who underperform at work before eventually retiring on ill health grounds (Alzheimer's Society 2019b). Early-onset dementia and employment were explored by Roach and Drummond (2014) who found that leaving work could be a traumatic and sudden event following diagnosis. Furthermore some families felt that their relative with dementia was treated unfairly and casually dismissed without proper consultation. They also highlighted that employers were liable to simply assume that job performance had slipped because of dementia without exploring other possible causes.

Evans (2019) explored the impact on people with young-onset dementia who were still working, describing their experiences from the onset of dementia-related symptoms until the time they left employment. Ten people with dementia were recruited (seven men and three women) from five Australian states. The average age of these people was 57 years, with ages ranging from 49 to 64 years. Four of these participants had Alzheimer's disease, three had fronto-temporal dementia and the other three had other types of dementia. Participants' experiences included the following:

- The emergence of dementia at work for the participants took the form of a slow transition that initially was not noticed by co-workers. It brought about subtle changes as the person became forgetful, disorganized, made mistakes and was slower.
- Over time the person's job performance continued to deteriorate and others at the workplace started to realize that there was a problem.
- Some were seen to be poor workers and so experienced difficulties with supervisors and co-workers. Others encountered difficulties managing changing relationships at work and negotiating the complex world of the workplace.
- Few were able to continue working beyond their diagnosis, and several raised concerns about the lack of opportunities for people who develop dementia while still employed.

One of the conclusions from the study highlighted that few of the participants were able to continue working beyond receiving their diagnosis and that there were concerns about a lack of opportunities for young people with dementia. This is strongly reflected within the social experiment showcased in the Channel 4 programme *The Restaurant That Makes Mistakes* (2019) with a group of people with dementia recruited to take on all of the required duties involved in running a restaurant. It appeared that most participants had previously lost confidence in their own abilities on account of the lowered expectations brought about by their diagnosis. The powerful impact of peer support and an environment that believed in and supported them brought about some striking results, including an enhanced well-being and significant improvement in cognitive ability. It also highlighted the continued productivity and contributions that can be made to the workforce by those with dementia.

A final thought within this section can be given to the concerns that families might have with the entrance of dementia into their midst, bringing with it the spectre of inheritance and the genetic link. We can consider here the worry that children might have regarding their future but also the burden of guilt, crushing anxiety and helplessness that the person with dementia is liable to feel contemplating what they are potentially passing on to their family. This is expressed by both Daniel (diagnosed with dementia in his thirties) and his wife in relation to their two-year-old twins and their 50–50 chance of inheriting the condition. We can also consider the connotations from a cultural context that a fear of genetic inheritance can have upon relationships. Lavis (2014) argued that some communities believe that the consequences of dementia will have an adverse impact on the family in terms of marriage prospects, particularly in communities where arranged marriage is prevalent. This is poignantly represented in the Indian drama film *Maine Gandhi Ko Nahin Mara* (*I Did Not Kill Gandhi*) about a retired professor with dementia with a particular scene showing a prospective marriage partner's family scared away by witnessing the father's erratic behaviour.

Initial follow-up support ('We are in need of information')

There is a wealth of evidence alerting us to the fact that following a dementia diagnosis families are in need of informational support (Ducharme *et al.* 2011; Fortinsky 2009). This is in relation to the many unanswered questions they might have as well as all of the questions they are still struggling to formulate. Essentially, people will be desirous of understanding what the condition of dementia actually entails, untangling the true facts from the wealth of misinformation and stigmatizing notions that abound. There is power and opportunities for personal autonomy through knowing and the provision of information facilitates autonomous approaches to continued dealing with daily living by those diagnosed with dementia and their families.

Gill's Narrative 3.3: Feeling lost

'When we were at the GP's getting a diagnosis, the doctor asked if we had any questions. Well, we were both in such shock and unable to think straight, let alone have any idea as to what it was we wanted to know. She did give us a stack of leaflets and a little booklet that I later retrieved from the bottom of my handbag and had a look through. I found them a little bewildering and hard to make sense of though. I did go back to the surgery and met with a nurse and

had an hour of her time, which helped greatly. I would have liked much more of her time as there is so much I need to talk about and make sense of. I was sent away with more bloody leaflets and lists of "helpful" organizations.

We have spent hours "getting lost" whilst trawling through numerous internet sites. I found news about treatments and interventions that could help Peter with his dementia as well as us as a family. I don't know though what to make of them. There were some wonderful sounding initiatives although nothing that we could realistically access. They seemed to be part of ongoing trials or initiatives being carried out in other countries. Peter had an awful time online and was getting so irritable and short-tempered that I had to urge him to go out for a walk. I think our web search has left us both more confused and hopeless.

What I would really like is to talk to a real expert, a "buddy" or guide. It would be useful to meet with someone who is in the same situation as us and able to properly understand what we are going through. They could give us a glimpse as to what the future has in store for us as well as what we can do to cope better.'

- *Could you recommend any websites that could be helpful for Gill?*
- *Do you know of any agencies/services where you live that offer support for people newly diagnosed and their family/partner?*

Gill's narrative reflects a process of information overload with her and Peter feeling progressively more lost and confused with each subsequent piece received. Her suggestion for a 'buddy' or 'guide' is a heartfelt plea for someone to assist them through this mind-boggling process. She mentions her and Peter being connected with others in a similar position who can provide meaningful and contextualized information. Meetings with practitioners can greatly assist although families may continue to have many of their questions unanswered, feeling confused or unable to properly articulate what they wish to say. What is being requested here is having access to people who it is felt intuitively understand and with whom one feels safe to explore feelings, no matter how painful or difficult they seem.

To begin with we might consider what families' informational needs might be, which, as advocated by Frenette and Beauchemin (2005), include details around the natural evolution of the disease, risk factors, power of attorney, driving, medical follow-up, risks of polypharmacy, resources for psychological support of caregivers and orientation to community resources (for helping patients remain at home). A first port of call for many confused and knowledge-hungry individuals after receiving a diagnosis of dementia is to turn to the internet. It can indeed be an extensive resource providing a wealth of up-to-the-minute information from numerous differing sites and perspectives (Morris 2006). Grassel *et al.* (2009) investigated the importance of the internet as a source of information for family caregivers of dementia patients and found it ranked fourth, behind doctors, counselling centres and related literature. It was found to be particularly significant for younger, better-educated family caregivers. As with other health themes the diversity can appear overwhelming with significant difficulties experienced in determining what the better or most appropriate sites might be. The need many people have following a dementia diagnosis is for understanding in order to allay anxieties and gain a clearer sense of what they are having to contend with. There will also be a need for answers as to how and why they ended up with dementia as well as a search for hope concerning available treatments and interventions. 'Wonder cures' and hopeful research studies or trials reported in their early stages will be eagerly reviewed for any help they can offer.

A problem with searching the internet for information relates to the sheer amount and diversity of what is available. A 2019 UK Google search carried out by the authors using the search term 'dementia' revealed a staggering 96 million sites. The first few accessible sites prominently included the UK's Alzheimer's Society and the US' Alzheimer's Association, two major organizations geared towards dementia support. The results will differ though depending upon what exactly is being searched for with additional terms such as 'causes', 'treatment', 'prognosis' or 'risk factors' all providing separate results. If wading through the list of sites indicated, one will soon notice the growing disparity in quality and informational types. As well as finding detailed and helpful information, individuals will also encounter a plethora of sites containing misleading or poorly organized resources as well as sponsored sites or advertisements promoting specific products and services. This even includes treatment offered for dementia in dogs with a whole industry prepared to sell products to consumers (e.g. canine services Spruce Pets or The Dog People). The sources or bodies offering websites vary in terms of credibility and expertise. There are, though, a range of reputable agencies accessible which include professional bodies, service-user and carer organizations and research groups. The *experts by experience* requested by Gill would provide a welcome resource and support whilst navigating the sea of dementia.

The varying types of informational resource are likely to produce different emotions in those searching for data. The early stages of dementia, for example, are outlined in an information sheet by the Alzheimer's Society (2007) highlighting the progressive nature of this disease:

> Often this phase is only apparent in hindsight and can be misattributed to bereavement, stress or normal ageing:
>
> - loss of short-term memory
> - loss of interest in hobbies and leisure activities
> - difficulty handling money
> - poor judgement
> - unwillingness to make decisions
> - difficulty in adapting to change
> - irritability/distress if unable to do something
> - repetitive questioning and loss of thread of conversation.

We can imagine that whilst helping to prepare families for the months and years ahead the contemplation of this range of difficulties could also prove disheartening and distressing. Their factsheet entitled 'After a Diagnosis', however, provides encouragement for those diagnosed with dementia to remain as independent as possible and urges them to continue to engage in their usual activities and occupations (Alzheimer's Society 2012). It also gives advice and support concerning future care options, financial and legal affairs, benefits, lasting powers of attorney, making a will, advance decisions, drugs for dementia, driving and working. Whilst some of the information here will be enormously helpful, contemplating the totality of themes can appear daunting and depressing. *Knowing* and *understanding*, though, can help individuals achieve a measure of consolation and feel better prepared. The need for education is also emphasized by the importance of challenging erroneous facts and understanding. There are a number of myths circulating about dementia among some BAME communities. This is largely to do with the negative connotations from associating dementia with mental illness, for example some black Caribbean people assumed that the mental illness was a result of a person being possessed by evil spirits and in the case of the Pakistani community possession by 'Jinns' (All Party Parliamentary Group on Dementia 2013).

ACTIVITY 3.5

How would you describe your cultural upbringing and do you feel this has influenced your understanding of dementia?

Do you feel there are merits, or not, in providing dementia education in schools, and why?

'Wonder cures'

We can imagine a search for information is in some cases carried out by individuals desperate for hope. Consider what their feelings might be when encountering so-called 'wonder cures' or reporting around potential innovations. The following list provides a sample taken from newspaper headlines and internet sites:

- 'Alzheimer's BREAKTHROUGH: Wonder drug moves step closer after undergoing human trials.' *Daily Express* (2017).
- 'Experts excited by brain "wonder-drug".' BBC (2017).
- 'Under-40s will never know misery of dementia as cure will be found "within two decades".' *The Telegraph* (2016).
- 'Are we really on the brink of a cure for Alzheimer's?' *The Guardian* (2018).
- 'My mum couldn't remember who I was – but then we changed her diet and her dementia improved.' *Cambridge News* (2018).
- 'Dementia breakthrough as new disease type identified.' *The Times* (2019).
- 'Dementia cure could be found in 5 years, world expert claims.' The Good Care Group (2019).

ACTIVITY 3.6

What do you think Gill and Peter would make of the listed headlines?

Do you feel headlines of this type are helpful, or not, and why?

Vernooij-Dassen *et al.* (2003) identified the need for information to extend beyond what clinicians considered relevant to also encompass the needs of patients and caregivers. Wackerbarth and Johnson (2002) noted that information concerning diagnosis and treatment as well as legal and financial issues was regarded as more important by family members than general information about the disease. They recommended that practitioners take note of caregivers' different informational and support needs and acknowledge that these needs could change throughout the caregiving experience. Sullivan, Muscat and Mulgrew (2007) investigated knowledge gaps and misconceptions about Alzheimer's disease and found the overall level of understanding to be quite poor. This in part reflects the findings from Gibson and Anderson's (2011) study with caregivers, indicating that they were inadequately informed about the condition of dementia or available community resources after diagnosis. The importance of properly informing and supporting caregivers is evidenced by Ducharme *et al.*'s (2011) research with those attending a psycho-educational individual programme being subsequently more knowledgeable and confident about their caring role, making more frequent use of the coping strategies of problem solving and reframing.

The disparity in informational needs is also experienced within families as evidenced by Edelman *et al.*'s (2006) study where individuals with Alzheimer's disease and family caregivers revealed substantial disagreement in terms of each partner's interest in information and services. Clearly, carers and families will have differing needs and Harland and Bath (2008) advocate the use of a user-centred informational approach to take account of individual needs. Millenaar *et al.* (2014) found that in addition to practical information, more accessible and specific information about the diagnosis and the course of young-onset dementia is needed to provide a better understanding of the disease for the children concerned. These findings underline the need for a personal, family-centred approach. We can also consider the findings from Baker *et al.*'s (2018) research with strong themes emerging of children needing to know the whole truth about dementia; that individuals with dementia are 'still people'; that it is 'not the fault' of the person with dementia; and that dementia is different and typically unpredictable for everyone. Discussions also indicated a need to educate children about ways to relate to a person with dementia, and to appreciate 'positives' within a relationship.

West and Bailey (2013) found that what was taught about dementia in schools within England was lacking in information. Isaac *et al.* (2017) evaluated adolescent knowledge and attitudes towards dementia. They invited 450 adolescents, aged 15–18 years, from schools across Sussex to complete a series of questions that assessed their dementia knowledge and attitudes. A total of 359 adolescent students completed the questionnaires.

Regarding the 15 questions relating to dementia knowledge, the participants were on average able to answer fewer than half correctly. Furthermore their responses to the attitudes questions showed students had both positive and negative attitudes towards dementia. The educational deficit reflected here is being tackled through various initiatives that are being rolled out in schools. In terms of the uptake of such programmes Farina (2017) surveyed teaching staff in 63 secondary schools (teaching ages 11–16) across East Sussex, West Sussex, and Brighton and Hove. The majority of participants expressed an interest in including some form of dementia education in the future. However, only nine schools currently had dementia education embedded in their curriculum and this was often part of broader topics in Personal, Social and Health Education. Furthermore only three schools had engaged with the annual Dementia Awareness Week.

Making sense ('Why me? Why us?')

The previous sections have explored the sense of shock and need for understanding following a diagnosis of dementia. Along with a family's support needs and enhanced understanding are likely to be requirements for finding answers to questions such as 'Why me?' or 'Why us?' This relates to potential causative or risk factors and will help to clarify whether individuals could have done anything to prevent the onset of dementia. This section explores a variety of related factors concerning a family's search for understanding.

Gill's Narrative 3.4: How has this occurred?

'Why has this happened to us, what have we done to deserve it? We have both worked hard all our lives, bringing up a family and should by rights now be expecting to enjoy some time together. It is just so unfair! Isn't dementia supposed to be an old person's illness? Peter's great-aunt had dementia although she was in her eighties and I don't recall anyone younger than about 70 in the care home. I have read somewhere about certain lifestyles causing risks. What was it about coffee or drinking wine? Were they protective or contributory factors?

What could we have done to prevent this happening? We have always eaten healthily and Peter regularly exercises although maybe he could have done more. He used to play football but that was some years ago now. Recently we watched a documentary about footballers and boxers who potentially developed dementia as a consequence of repeated impact to the head. Could heading the ball have contributed towards this? He had smoked for many years before switching to vaping. Could that be a factor? I did keep on at him about how harmful it was for his health although he wouldn't listen. Why didn't he take his health more seriously?'

- *Do you find yourself agreeing with some or all of Gill's thoughts?*
- *What advice or support could you offer Gill during this emotionally turbulent time?*

Gill's narrative shows her searching for answers, moving between various risk factors but without any solace being found. This is in part generated through the impact of the diagnosis and the need for hope. Allen, Oyebode and Allen (2009, p.477) concluded that the: 'confluence of young-onset dementia and the stage of development of these young people appear to produce a response in which grief, perceived threat and isolation are central features'.

The sense of shock will engage many questions including how this could have occurred or what might have been done differently to have avoided it. The search for clues will cover biological, psychological and social considerations with key aspects such as predisposing characteristics, lifestyle factors or attention upon the genetic base. The soul-searching following a diagnosis of dementia, especially in the case of young-onset dementia, is likely to involve an examination of risk factors. The purpose of this is to gain a better understanding as to how this could have happened as well as the potentially torturous and guilt-laden process of wondering whether it could have been anticipated or avoided.

There are likely to be some very polarized emotions evoked through observing some of the thought-provoking or alarmist newspaper headlines. Arguably their messages are succinct and certainly eye-catching, and appear to encourage their readership to become fearful and uncertain (see Activity 3.7).

ACTIVITY 3.7: NEWS REPORTING OF DEMENTIA RISK FACTORS

- 'People who suffer from cold sores are more likely to develop Alzheimer's disease' *The Daily Telegraph* (2 November 2007)
- 'Obesity doubles the risk of Alzheimer's' *Daily Express* (8 May 2008)

- 'A fatty acid, an ingredient found in foods considered healthy, could harm brain cells and raise the risk of getting Alzheimer's disease' *The Guardian* (20 October 2008)
- 'Britain's long working hours could be putting millions at risk of dementia' *Daily Mail* (26 February 2009)
- 'Having depression may nearly double the risk of developing dementia later in life' BBC News (7 July 2010)
- 'Heavy smoking in mid-life more than doubles the risk of developing Alzheimer's disease' *The Independent* (26 October 2010)
- 'Long-term exposure to pesticides leads to greater risk of dementia' *The Independent* (2 December 2010)
- 'Scientists have discovered five gene variants that raise the risk of Alzheimer's disease' *The Guardian* (4 April 2011)
- 'Early-onset Alzheimer's strikes families fast and ferociously' BBC News Magazine (30 May 2012)
- 'General anaesthetic for over 65s raises risk of dementia by 35%' *Daily Mail* (1 June 2013)
- 'Third of dementia cases are preventable through nine life style changes, say researchers' *The Independent* (20 July 2017)

What emotions do you think these headlines generate?

Have you recently seen similar headlines and what were your thoughts?

If we consider Gill's present situation in trying to make sense of Peter's diagnosis, the headlines featured here may not be very helpful. Indeed, Thomas DeBaggio (2002, p.68), who was diagnosed with dementia, reflected: 'I get very angry when I hear someone talk about this disease as if it were brought on by improper diet or behaviour.'

Public Health England (2017) reviewed mid-life risk factors of dementia and focused on recent literature on the relationship between changes in risk factor behaviours or conditions in mid-life (ages 40 to 64) and onset of dementia later in life.

They found around one-third of cases of dementia in old age could potentially be prevented through changes in behaviour in mid-life (Norton *et al.* 2014). This highlights the importance of pursuing preventative measures, especially with the evidence that physical inactivity, smoking, diabetes, hypertension and obesity increase the risk of dementia.

However, if you add up the percentage risk of all the factors (some 35%) it still leaves some 65 per cent of factors outside the person's control, for example their age and family history. Huntley *et al.* (2017) published results on an online assessment of risk factors of 14,201 'non-demented individuals aged >50 years' by the use of four cognitive performance tasks online. They concluded that there were several potentially modifiable risk factors that could significantly contribute to cognitive performance. Higher educational achievement, the presence of a close confiding relationship and moderate alcohol intake were associated with benefits across all four cognitive tasks, and exercise was associated with better performance on verbal reasoning. A diagnosis of depression was negatively associated with performance on short-term memory. Also a history of stroke was negatively associated with verbal reasoning.

The Lancet Commission (2017) comprised a panel of 24 experts on dementia prevention, intervention and care and generated evidence-based recommendations included restricted educational opportunities; hearing loss and associated stress; lack of exercise and physical activity; hypertension, type 2 diabetes and obesity; smoking and cardiovascular conditions; depression; and a lack of social contact and isolation.

The Alzheimer's Society (2016a) provide a factsheet outlining the risk factors for dementia. These include age and genetics, but also medical conditions and lifestyle choices:

- ageing – strongest known risk factor for dementia
- gender – women are more likely to develop Alzheimer's disease than men whereas the position is reversed with vascular dementia
- ethnicity – South Asian people and people of African or African-Caribbean origin appear more predisposed to developing dementia
- genetics – having a close relative (parent or sibling) with Alzheimer's disease increases chances of developing the disease
- medical conditions/diseases – cardiovascular factors, type 2 diabetes, high blood pressure or blood cholesterol levels, obesity and head injury
- lifestyle – physical inactivity, smoking or excessive alcohol consumption.

One of the factors listed here is excessive alcohol consumption. Alcohol causes damage to the brain in a number of different ways including direct toxicity to brain cells, an interference with thiamine absorption in the brain and associated vascular damage (Cox, Anderson and McCabe 2004). Sachdeva *et al.*'s (2016) review study recognizes the term 'alcohol-induced persisting dementia' as progressive intellectual and cognitive decline where aphasia (absence of previously acquired language skills), apraxia (difficulties in undertaking motor activities) and agnosia (failure to recognize or identify objects) can be experienced. Furthermore the person may have memory impairments impacting upon new learning and the recall of previously learnt information. Gupta and Warner (2008, p.352) posit that this century will witness a silent epidemic of alcohol-related dementia: 'Given the neurotoxic effects of alcohol and the inexorable increase in per capita consumption, future generations may see a disproportionate increase in alcohol-related dementia.'

McCabe (2011, p.163) concludes that there is evidence to suggest that:

> Muddying the water further is the stigma associated with alcohol problems, with dementia and with ageing. At the moment there are many people drinking over recommended limits who do not recognize their behaviour as harmful, focusing instead on problems such as binge drinking which they see as distinct from themselves.

This serves to underline one of the number of lifestyle 'choices' that people might be engaged in which singly or collectively contribute towards an increased risk of later developing dementia.

Telling others ('Who should we tell? What can we say?')

Sharing information about an individual's diagnosis might be delayed or maybe avoided given the feared connotations. Keith Oliver (2019, p.51), diagnosed with dementia in his fifties, recalls telling colleagues about his potential diagnosis: 'Never have I seen a group of people in the collective, stunned hush that blanketed the classroom we were in. I could not speak afterwards and left silently.'

Revealing a dementia diagnosis will evidently be very hard, influenced by who the person is and the likely consequences such as causing upset, engaging stigma or evoking restrictions. Telling children, for example, or other family members is likely to be carried out extremely hesitantly. The thought, for example, 'How do you tell a young child their dad has dementia' can seem crippling and seemingly impossible to act upon. The stigmatizing element is fuelled by lowered societal expectations of those with dementia and may be very keenly felt within various cultural groups. Finally, the imparting of information about a dementia diagnosis can have profound ramifications within the workplace with colleagues and employers questioning one's ability to remain in the workplace.

Gill's Narrative 3.5: Telling people

'We are in a bit of a dilemma as to what to do about telling people about Peter's diagnosis. Who do you tell? When is the best time? What do you actually say to them? The children are aware of their dad's diagnosis now and it was absolutely horrible having to tell them. Ashleigh I think wasn't really surprised. Matt didn't really respond much to this news. Tom though I am especially worried about. At first he questioned me about it but since then has been very quiet and withdrawn. You should never have to tell a young boy that his dad has dementia. What do I say to Peter's mother? I know she lives in a nursing home now but she's not confused. She gets very anxious and phones us every day. How on earth do I tell her that her son has dementia? It will totally destroy her.

Peter's condition is getting worse and the changes are certainly more apparent to me. Those only having casual contact with Peter, though, might put his erratic behaviour down to stress or tiredness. I feel very mixed about talking to people outside of the family and Tina, our immediate neighbour, comes to mind. She gave me a hug and kept repeating how awful it was although it felt very awkward and I got the impression that she was relieved when she could eventually get away. Since then, I have had little contact with her and she always seems too busy to stop and chat which I suppose suits both of us.

And then there is Peter's workplace. He has been signed off work for a while on health grounds but that was when the GP diagnosed depression. If we tell them, will he be able to stay there? If we don't, what problems is he likely to experience?'

- *If you were Gill, what conversations might you have with Matt about Dad?*
- *If you were Gill, what conversations might you have with Tom about Dad?*
- *Do you have an opinion on how an employer may view an employee with a diagnosis of dementia?*

Gill's narrative and your responses to the suggested questions highlight the dilemma faced by individuals following a dementia diagnosis, namely decisions around who to tell, when to divulge information and what to actually say. We can consider perhaps how different it feels when confiding such difficult and emotive news to children, partners, siblings, parents, friends, neighbours or work colleagues. Issues here include worries around causing distress, being met with disbelief, feelings of shame or stigmatization and implications with regard to the workplace.

Divulging information to those outside of the immediate family can sometimes be met with direct opposition or an unwillingness to acknowledge the presence of dementia. Jackson (2010) recalls that in the early days following her husband's diagnosis, visitors often doubted that there was anything wrong. It is especially hard for others to acknowledge or understand what the problems might be, especially with a condition that in the earlier stages may be hard to detect. Individuals can appear lucid and at this stage are unlikely to fit the stereotypical view of frail and markedly confused people. Indeed, Christine Bryden (2005), a very eloquent speaker and writer on the topic of dementia, has at times struggled to convince others that she has the condition, feeling compelled to show pictures of her own brain scans. In fact, her recent MRI brain scan picture is included on her website and she remarks that if only people could see the visible brain damage, they would actively cheer the dementia survivors (Bryden 2015b). This is a telling statement, allowing us indeed to cheer on and celebrate the notable achievements of those living with and coping with marked cognitive deterioration. The emphasis changes from what individuals *are no longer able* to do to what they *are still able* to do.

Terry Pratchett (2015) observed: 'It is a strange life, when you "come out". People get embarrassed, lower their voices, get lost for words.'

Unsurprisingly many people will struggle with making their diagnosis known and in some cases will attempt to conceal it. The following case study is taken from research by Husband (1999) examining the psychological consequences of learning a diagnosis of dementia:

> He was angry about the diagnosis and tended to think he had to be 'on his guard' the whole time in case he 'gave himself away'. This hypervigilance was exhausting and made him irritable. He believed that if people knew he had dementia they would laugh at him, and watch to see if he made a fool of himself.

Telling other people about a dementia diagnosis might be avoided because of this perceived stigma and lowered expectations from others. Indeed the negative perceptions associated with a dementia diagnosis are highlighted by the results of the Alzheimer's Society's canvassing in May 2018 of over

2000 members of the general public about their perceptions of dementia. Their findings indicated that people with dementia:

- can be unpredictable (68%)
- should not be allowed to drive (60%)
- experience discrimination (56%)
- should not go on holiday on their own (50%)
- should not be left alone (47%)
- need constant supervision (39%)
- could live on their own (29%)
- are likely to be violent (25%)
- are not able to continue working (19%).

ACTIVITY 3.8

If you are a health or social care practitioner, do you feel the negative perceptions outlined can have an influence on the ways you work?

If you work in either a single or multi-professional team have you experienced negative perceptions? If so, how were these issues addressed?

Whilst it might be anticipated that the process of telling others can be met by unhelpful responses it is important to consider the support that can be realized through relating information to others. An interviewee in the Healthtalk (2019) website related:

> I was always very open with it, with all our friends…as a result they knew how to react. I ended up amazed at the fact that I had sixteen volunteers I could call on. And they were marvellous, they came and they all knew my wife.

It is refreshing to note the positive responses received here with the *sixteen volunteers* clearly an immense level of reassurance for this interviewee and his wife. What though of the process involved when telling relatives? Gill's narrative highlights the difficulties involved regarding who to tell and what to tell them. Of particular concern was her worry about the impact upon their children with special worry about the youngest, Tom. The Alzheimer's Society (2017) booklet 'Young-Onset Dementia: Understanding Your Diagnosis' appreciates parents' desire to protect their children yet stresses the importance of talking with them as they are likely to be aware that something is occurring and needing to know that it is not because of them. They highlight the need to allow children to come to terms with a parent's diagnosis in their own time and to maintain an ongoing dialogue with them. Similarly, their booklet 'Explaining Dementia to Children and Young People' (Alzheimer's Society 2016b) stresses that young children are likely to be aware of tensions in the family and advises on ways of including them. Diana Friel McGowin (1993) recalled gathering her family together to tell them about her diagnosis. She recalls her news being met with quiet stoicism and acceptance. Similarly, Htay (2010), although wanting to protect family members, decided to tell them right from the start. This resulted in personal support and a reduction in his overall burden of caring. A key issue with telling other people about a family member's diagnosis is the concern that the term 'dementia' will overshadow the person and drain them of their perceived capabilities. This is reinforced through commonly attributed notions of dementia as a hopeless, debilitating condition.

A progressively ageing population and the growing number of people with young-onset dementia means that having to tell parents (and potentially grandparents) about their adult children having dementia need not be uncommon. An interviewee on the Healthtalk (2019) site relates how difficult and distressing this was:

> [A] very bad moment was when I had to tell his mother who was in her eighties, that [my husband] had got Alzheimer's. I'd pussy-foot around a bit because she was a terrible worrier...having to tell her I think was a horrible moment because I think your child suffering with dementia must be almost worse than having your spouse, because still, you still see them as so much younger. Time and again she said 'I wish I could change places with him.' That was a nasty moment; it really was.

This highlights all too clearly the family member's anguish at considering how to tell her husband's elderly mother about his diagnosis.

How true could this be today?

The theme of 'How true could this be today?' asks you to consider reframing an observation from the past. This commentary had an influence in informing thinking at that time whilst also determining opinions of the day. A number of questions will encourage you to consider its relevance in the here and now, such as: have national opinions changed or not? Do you agree or not with these comments? What has influenced your attitudes?

Background information: Goffman's research interests had a focus on psychiatric stigma; however, he did comment that the differences between a normal and stigmatized person was a question of perspective, not reality, and that stigma is in the eye of the beholder. Stigma was undesirable, 'a trait deeply discrediting' with attributes that 'disqualify one from full social acceptance' (1963, p.1).

- Do you agree or not with these observations from the 1960s?
- Do you think that a diagnosis of dementia carries certain expectations for the individual and their family/friends?
- Do you believe that public awareness of individuals with dementia is 'stigma free'?
- What evidence have you for the above responses?

Concluding thoughts

This chapter began by inviting you to accompany Gill, Peter and their family on the ways they were making sense post-diagnosis by moving from coping with shock, through the questioning of 'Why us?' to the position of telling others. As a 'family member' (and as a friend) you have been able to access regular updates courtesy of Gill's narratives and have been encouraged to get closer to the lived and felt experiences. Your responses to the various activities reflect both your personal and probable societal perceptions on what receiving a diagnosis of dementia can mean for the individual and significant other people in their lives. The next part of the Lawrence family journey covers the ways that the family members contemplate the commencement with their journey as a person, couple or family with dementia.

PERSONAL LEARNING

What was your past knowledge and understanding, what new learning have you achieved and how could this inform your future personal and/or professional interventions?

As a 'family member', my new learning includes ....

....

On reading the first-person narratives, my new learning includes

....

INTERVENTIONS

Be mindful that whatever comments are offered should be realistic, achievable and person-centred. Also that the feelings conveyed and observations made reinforce that 'making sense was now paramount' for the individual and significant other people in their life.

The types of interventions could include ....

....

References

All Party Parliamentary Group on Dementia (2013). *Dementia Does Not Discriminate: The Experience of Black Asian and Minority Ethnic Communities.* Accessed on 2/12/17 at www.alzheimers.org.uk/2013-appg-report.

Allen, J., Oyebode, J. and Allen, J. (2009). 'Having a father with young-onset dementia: the impact on well-being of young people.' *The International Journal of Social Research and Practice* 8, 4, 455–480.

Alzheimer's Society (2007). *Information Sheet: The Progression of Dementia.* London: Alzheimer's Society.

Alzheimer's Society (2012). *Factsheet: After a Diagnosis.* Accessed on 10/7/17 at www.alzheimers.org.uk/site/scripts/documents_info.php?documentID=122.

Alzheimer's Society (2016a). *Factsheet 450LP: Risk Factors for Dementia.* Accessed on 12/11/19 at www.alzheimers.org.uk/sites/default/files/pdf/factsheet_risk_factors_for_dementia.pdf.

Alzheimer's Society (2016b). *Explaining Dementia to Children and Young People.* Accessed on 16/5/17 at www.alzheimers.org.uk/sites/default/files/migrate/downloads/factsheet_explaining_dementia_to_children_and_young_people.pdf.

Alzheimer's Society (2017). *Young-Onset Dementia: Understanding Your Diagnosis.* Accessed on 10/5/18 at www.alzheimers.org.uk/sites/default/files/migrate/downloads/young-onset_dementia_understanding_your_diagnosis.pdf.

Alzheimer's Society (2018). *Dementia-Friendly Media and Broadcast Guide.* London: Alzheimer's Society.

Alzheimer's Society (2019a). *Mum Diagnosed Today at 54.* Accessed on 31/1/20 at https://forum.alzheimers.org.uk/threads/mum-diagnosed-today-at-54.118060.

Alzheimer's Society (2019b). *Within Three Months of My Diagnosis I Lost My Job and got Depression.* Accessed on 10/11/19 at www.alzheimers.org.uk/blog/chris-story-unemployed-after-diagnosis.

Aminzadeh F., Byszewski A., Molnar, F.J. and Eisner, M. (2007). 'Emotional impact of dementia diagnosis: exploring persons with dementia and caregivers' perspectives.' *Aging and Mental Health 11* (3), 281–290.

Baker, J., Jeon,Y., Goodenough, B. and Low, L. (2018). 'What do children need to know about dementia? The perspectives of children and people with personal experience of dementia.' *International Psychogeriatrics 30* (5), 673–684.

Barua, Jahnu (dir.) (2005). *I Did Not Kill Gandhi* [Film]. India: Curtain Call Co.

BBC One (2019). *Our Dementia Choir with Vicky McClure.* 2 May.

Bryden, C. (2005). *Dancing with Dementia.* London: Jessica Kingsley Publishers.

Bryden, C. (2015a). *Nothing About Us, Without Us! 20 Years of Dementia Advocacy.* London: Jessica Kingsley Publishers.

Bryden, C. (2015b). *Christine Bryden.* Accessed 12/12/19 at www.christinebryden.com/christine-now.

Bryden, C. (2018). *Will I Still Be Me? Finding a Continuing Sense of Self in the Lived Experience of Dementia.* London: Jessica Kingsley Publishers.

Channel 4 (2019). *The Restaurant That Makes Mistakes.* 12 June.

Chaplin, R. and Davidson, I. (2016). 'What are the experiences of people with dementia in employment?' *Dementia 15* (2), 147–161.

Clare, L., Wilson, B., Carter, G., Breen, K., Berrios, G. and Hodges, J. (2002). 'Depression and anxiety in memory clinic attenders and their carers: implications for evaluating the effectiveness of cognitive rehabilitation interventions.' *International Journal of Geriatric Psychiatry 17*, 962–967.

Clemerson, G., Walsh, S. and Isaac, C. (2014). 'Towards living with young-onset dementia: an exploration of coping from the perspective of those diagnosed.' *The International Journal of Social Research and Practice 13* (4), 451–466.

Connell, C. Roberts, J., McLaughlin, S. and Carpenter, B. (2009). 'Black and white adult family members' attitudes toward a dementia diagnosis.' *Journal of the American Geriatrics Society 57* (9), 1562–1568.

Cox, S., Anderson, I. and McCabe, L. (2004). *A Fuller Life: Report of the Expert Group on Alcohol Related Brain Damage*. Edinburgh: Scottish Executive.

DeBaggio, T. (2002). *Losing My Mind: An Intimate Look at Alzheimer's*. New York: The Free Press.

Department of Health (2009). *National Dementia Strategy*. London: HMSO.

De Vugt, M. and Verhey, F. (2013). 'The impact of early dementia diagnosis and intervention on informal caregivers.' *Progress in Neurobiology 110*, 54–62.

Draper, B., Peisah, C., Snowdon, J. and Brodaty, H. (2009). 'Early dementia diagnosis and the risk of suicide and euthanasia.' *Alzheimer's and Dementia 6* (1), 75–82.

Draper, B. and Withall, A. (2016). 'Young onset dementia.' *International Medicine Journal 46* (7), 779–786.

Ducharme, F., Levesque, L., Lachance, L., Kergoat, M., Legault, A., Beaudet, M. and Zarit, S. (2011). 'Learning to become a family caregiver: efficacy of an intervention program for caregivers following diagnosis of dementia in a relative.' *Gerontologist 51* (4), 484–489.

Edelman, P., Kuhn, D., Fulton, B. and Kyrouac, G. (2006). 'Information and service needs of persons with Alzheimer's disease and their family caregivers living in rural communities.' *American Journal of Alzheimer's Disease and Other Dementias 21* (4), 226–233.

Evans, D. (2019). 'An exploration of the impact of young onset dementia on employment.' *Dementia 18* (1), 262–281.

Farina, N. (2017). 'What is taught about dementia in secondary schools? A survey of schools in Sussex, England.' *Dementia 0* (0), 1–9.

Fortinsky, R. (2009). 'Diagnosis and early support.' In M. Downs and B. Bowers (eds) *Excellence in Dementia Care: Research into Practice*. London: McGraw Hill.

Frenette, G. and Beauchemin, J. (2005). 'Sad but true: your father has dementia. An approach to announcing the diagnosis.' *Canadian Family Physician 49* (Oct.), 1296–1301.

Friel McGowin, D. (1993). *Living in the Labyrinth: A Personal Journey Through the Maze of Alzheimer's*. New York: Delacorte Press.

Gibson, A. and Anderson, K. (2011). 'Difficult diagnoses: family caregivers' experiences during and following the diagnostic process for dementia.' *American Journal of Alzheimer's Disease and Other Dementias 26* (3), 212–217.

Gillies, A. (2009). *Keeper: A Book about Memory, Identity, Isolation*. London: Short Books.

Goffman, E. (1963). *Stigma: Notes on the Management of Spoiled Identity*. Harmondsworth: Penguin.

Grassel, E., Bleich, S., Meyer-Wegener, K., Schmid, U., Kornhuber, J. and Prokosch, H. (2009). 'Das Internet als Informationsquelle fur pflegende Angehorige eines Demenzpatienten.' *Psychiatrische Praxis 36* (3), 115–118.

Gupta, S. and Warner, J. (2008). 'Alcohol-related dementia: a 21st century silent epidemic?' *The British Journal of Psychiatry 193*, 351–353.

Harland, J. and Bath, P. (2008). 'Understanding the information behaviours of carers of people with dementia: a critical review of models from information science.' *Aging & Mental Health 12* (4), 467–477.

Harris, P. (2004). 'The perspective of younger people with dementia: still an overlooked population.' *Social Work in Mental Health 2* (4), 17–36.

Healthtalk (2019). *Carers of People with Dementia – Friends and Family*. Accessed on 31/1/20 at https://healthtalk.org/carers-people-dementia/friends-and-family.

Htay, U. (2010). 'We learn to enter her world.' In L. Whitman (ed.) *Telling Tales About Dementia: Experiences of Caring*. London: Jessica Kingsley Publishers.

Huntley, J., Corbett, A., Wesness, K., Hampshire, A. and Bollard, C. (2017). 'Risk factors for dementia and cognitive function in healthy adults.' *Alzheimer's and Dementia 13* (7), 1194–1195.

Husband, H. (1999). 'The psychological consequences of learning a diagnosis of dementia: three case examples.' *Aging and Mental Health 3* (2), 179–183.

Innes, A., Szymczynska, P. and Stark, C. (2014). 'Dementia diagnosis and post-diagnostic support in Scottish rural communities: experiences of people with dementia and their families.' *Dementia 13* (2), 233–247.

Isaac, M., Isaac, M., Farina, N. and Tabet, N. (2017). 'Knowledge and attitudes towards dementia in adolescent students.' *Journal of Mental Health 26* (5), 419–425.

Jackson, D. (2010). 'The most difficult decision in my life.' In L. Whitman (ed.) *Telling Tales About Dementia: Experiences of Caring*. London: Jessica Kingsley Publishers.

Lancet Commission (2017). *Dementia Prevention, Intervention, and Care*. Accessed on 4/7/18 at www.thelancet.com/commissions/dementia2017.

Lavis, P. (2014). 'The Importance of Promoting Mental Health in Children and Young People from Black and Minority Ethnic Communities.' *Better Health Briefing 33*. London: Race Equality Foundation.

McCabe, L. (2011). 'Alcohol, ageing and dementia: a Scottish perspective.' *Dementia 10* (2), 149–163.

Millenaar, J., Vliet, D., Bakker, C., Vernooij-Dassen, M., Koopmans, R., Verhey, F. and de Vugt, M. (2014). 'The experiences and needs of children living with a parent with young onset dementia: results from the NeedYD study.' *International Psychogeriatrics 26* (12), 2001–2010.

Moniz-Cook, E., Manthorpe, J., Carr, I., Gibson, G. and Vernooij-Dassern, M. (2006). 'Facing the future: a qualitative study of older people referred to a memory clinic prior to assessment and diagnosis.' *Dementia 5*, 375–395.

Morris, G. (2006). *Mental Health Issues and the Media*. London: Routledge.

Morris, G. and Morris, J. (2010). *The Dementia Care Workbook*. Buckingham: Open University Press.

Norton, S., Mathews, F., Barnes, D., Yaffe, K. and Brayne, C. (2014). 'Potential for primary prevention of Alzheimer's disease. An analysis of population-based data.' *Lancet Neurology 13* (8), 788–794.

Nurock, S. (2010). 'Look back in anger.' In L. Whitman (ed.) *Telling Tales About Dementia: Experiences of Caring*. London: Jessica Kingsley Publishers.

Oliver, K. (2019). *Dear Alzheimer's: A Diary of Living with Dementia*. London: Jessica Kingsley Publishers.

Pratchett, T. (2015). '"A butt of my own jokes": Terry Pratchett on the disease that finally claimed him.' Accessed on 7/8/16 at www.theguardian.com/books/2015/mar/15/a-butt-of-my-own-jokes-terry-pratchett-on-the-disease-that-finally-claimed-him.

Prince, M., Wimo, A., Guerchet, M., Ali, G., Wu, Y. and Prina, M. (2015). *World Alzheimer Report 2015. The Global Impact of Dementia: An Analysis of Prevalence, Incidence, Cost and Trends*. London: Alzheimer's Disease International.

Public Health England (2017). *The Effects of Mid-Life Risk Factors on Dementia. Key Messages*. Accessed on 7/8/18 at www.gov.uk/phe.

Roach, P. and Drummond, N. (2014). '"It's nice to have something to do": early-onset dementia and maintaining purposeful activity.' *Journal of Psychiatric and Mental Health Nursing 21*, 889–895.

Robinson, H. (2010). 'Glimpses of Glory on a Long, Grey Road.' In L. Whitman (ed.) *Telling Tales About Dementia: Experiences of Caring*. London: Jessica Kingsley Publishers.

Sachdeva, A., Chandra, M., Choudhary, M., Dayal, P. and Singh A. (2016). 'Alcohol-related dementia and neurocognitive impairment: a review study.' *International Journal of High Risk Behaviour Addiction 5* (3), e27976.

Spruce Pets (n.d.). *Dementia and Senility in Dogs*. Accessed on 17/9/18 at www.thesprucepets.com/dementia-in-dogs-1117412.

Stokes, L., Combes, H. and Stokes, G. (2014). 'Understanding the dementia diagnosis: the impact on the caregiving experience.' *Dementia 13* (1), 59–78.

Sullivan, K., Muscat, T. and Mulgrew, K. (2007). 'Knowledge of Alzheimer's disease among patients, carers, and noncarer adults: misconceptions, knowledge gaps, and correct beliefs.' *Topics in Geriatric Rehabilitation: Function and Cognition 23* (2), 137–148.

Svanberg, E., Spector, A. and Stott J. (2011). 'The impact of young-onset dementia on the family: a literature review.' *International Psychogeriatrics 23* (3), 356–371.

Swaffer, K. (2016). *What the Hell Happened to My Brain? Living Beyond Dementia*. London: Jessica Kingsley Publishers.

Swift, J. (2010). 'The Departing Light.' In L. Whitman (ed.) *Telling Tales About Dementia: Experiences of Caring*. London: Jessica Kingsley Publishers.

The Dog People (n.d.). *Dog Dementia: What Are the Symptoms and Treatment?* Accessed on 17/9/18 at www.rover.com/blog/canine-cognitive-dysfunction-major-symptoms.

Vernooij-Dassen, M., Van Hout, H., Hund, K., Hoefnagels, W. and Grol, R. (2003). 'Information for dementia patients and their caregivers: what information does a memory clinic pass on, and to whom?' *Aging and Mental Health 7* (1), 34–38.

Wackerbarth, S. and Johnson, M. (2002). 'Essential information and support needs of family caregivers.' *Patient Education and Counseling 47* (2), 95–100.

Waddell, G. and Burton, A. (2006). *Is Work Good for your Health and Wellbeing?* London: Department for Work and Pensions.

West, A. and Bailey, E. (2013). 'The development of the academies programme: "privatising" school-based education in England 1986–2013.' *British Journal of Educational Studies 61* (2), 137–159.

Young Dementia UK (2019). *Ken H's Story*. Accessed on 15/8/19 at www.youngdementiauk.org/ken-hs-story.

Zubatsky, M. (2015). 'Collaborative interventions for Alzheimer's caregivers following a family member's initial diagnosis. Alzheimer's and Dementia.' Conference: Alzheimer's Association International Conference 2015. Washington, DC, US. Conference Publication. 11 (7 Supplement 1), 461.

Chapter 4

Commencing the Dementia Journey

Introduction

This chapter examines a family's experiences when commencing their dementia journey. Whilst technically the journey described here can be regarded as having started at the point when first signs became evident (or even before that), the emphasis within this chapter is upon the conscious preparation for the coming years and the contemplation of living with the presence of *dementia* in the family. A key factor here involves the challenges of acknowledgement and acceptance of 'I have dementia' or 'We are a family with dementia'. Such recognition will pose obstacles and difficulties given the generally low expectations evoked when considering the condition of dementia. A central element engaged in by those concerned is *role transition* with each family member faced with having to make significant changes in order to preserve the continuing functioning of the family as a unit. For the person with dementia, worries are likely to centre on their growing dependency upon others as well as living with a steadily advancing *condition*, one commonly associated with high levels of pessimism and fear. For a number of people this heralds what they might regard as the commencement of their *illness journey*, an experience that affects individuals in very different ways across a spectrum from stoic acceptance to absolute despair. A partner or spouse will be faced with the contemplation of their loved one's decreasing independence and the expectation of taking on a future caring role, which poses challenges for their identity as a couple. There are further implications for younger carers, especially those in employment and with dependent children, having to consider what this means for their lives. The impact upon other family members includes the requirement to mentally recalibrate their concept of *family* and acceptance of the presence of dementia within their midst. For children and adolescents this will be especially confusing as they can be faced with a reversal of roles providing a 'parental' role for their own parents.

> ***The story so far***
>
> *Gill, Peter and their children are at the stage of contemplating their future individually and as a family group. The implications of Peter's dementia diagnosis are beginning to sink in with family members struggling with questions of 'Why me?' and 'Why us?' They have begun seeking answers to these questions through engaging with the healthcare services on offer and, as could be expected, conducting a fairly extensive internet search. Peter now has the prospect of seeking acceptance for his transition from mental well-health to mental ill-health, and the recognition of being a person with dementia. The implications for Gill involve the contemplation of having to make major adjustments in her life and potentially having to give up her employment in order to become a carer for her husband. Their children, having learned of their father's dementia, now have to consider what this means for them as a family and the prospect of maybe having to help care for their father.*

Chapter themes

The changing relationships within the family structure were prominently featured in Harris and Keady's (2009) study of the experience of early-onset dementia. These issues are central to this chapter's focus in terms of the journey commenced by a family when one of its members is diagnosed with dementia. This diagnosis can be seen here as being given not just to the individual undergoing organic brain changes but essentially to whole families. The ramifications will touch each person in their attempt to make sense of and acknowledge the meaning of having the presence of *dementia* as a condition or illness within their family. Themes within this chapter will focus in turn upon the perspective of different family members, and the associated narratives will accordingly address all parties:

- Person with dementia: beginning the illness journey – 'I have a condition'
- Partner/carer: on becoming a carer – 'We are a couple with dementia'
- Children/family members: role transitions – 'We are a family with dementia'

Person with dementia: beginning the illness journey ('I have a condition')

In keeping with the theme being addressed here, we are making a diversion from Gill's narratives and providing you with some of Peter's thoughts.

Peter's Narrative 4.1: Wavering emotions

'I do feel myself wavering between two positions – terrible despondency and hopelessness on one side and a determination to fight this condition, making the most of the life I have left on the other. My emotions and feelings are simply all over the place at this moment in time and I am finding it hard to take in what has happened. "Dementia", a reasonably straightforward word although one that seems so damning. I liken it to a bomb that has been thrown into our lives leaving us shell-shocked, battered and literally torn apart. I know things will never be the same although the extent of the devastation will only become apparent in time. At the moment I don't feel able to appreciate the full extent of the changes that this diagnosis will have on me. I feel cheated of my "healthy" years and the future now seems much harder to picture. Will dementia rob me of my feelings for Gill and the kids? Will I be able to keep up contact with friends? What about the community groups I am part of? Thoughts about my health and well-being are becoming all-consuming during the day and are creeping into my thoughts at night as well, preventing me from sleeping. I can look after myself at the moment, but what does the future hold?'

■ *One can only wonder what Peter could be feeling as he contemplates a different life with dementia. You may consider Peter's new life changes by considering factors that create a:*

- *positive impact on Peter's well-being*
- *negative impact on Peter's well-being.*

Peter's narrative expresses the polarized extent of his thoughts and feelings, moving between pessimistic despondency and courageous determination to meet the challenges ahead of him. Such a position is echoed in many narratives by people diagnosed with dementia, as shown in the following narrative:

> Like Columbus, I am on a voyage of discovery. My route is not exact and I must make adjustments as I go along...unlike being at sea in a storm, I know that the voyage is only going to become more difficult. It may become a typhoon or hurricane, depending on where it takes me. This storm will not

> pass: I have to make suitable preparations before the force 12 hits. Let me tell you that I am lucky: I have very good friends who will be with me on the stormy ride ahead. (Voyager 2005, cited in Morris and Morris 2010, p.17).

Voyager's narrative illustrates the sense that this is largely a journey into the unknown with difficult and tempestuous encounters anticipated. There is an expectation of hardship as well as the desire for continued anchoring and grounding by trusted companions. This narrative illustrates the acknowledgement of a journey (or voyage) commencing. It is however regarded here as a process of *discovery*, a term that anticipates new growth and learning. Indeed, this can be reflected against Kate Swaffer's (2016) positivistic notion of *living beyond dementia* or the recognition of a person's new identity emerging through the dementia process. There is contrast provided by other words and phrases in Voyager's narrative that employ weather metaphors to symbolize anticipated difficulty. The available evidence shows that the dementia journey can and does include examples of both polarized elements covered above. It is, however, a very individual journey with each person or family encountering their own unique set of experiences that include a mixture of components along the spectrum between points of despair and hope.

A point of significance, as raised by Peter, is the transition between states of health and illness and the recognition of self as a person with a *condition*. Such a transformation or metamorphosis takes the person between positions of *person without dementia* to *person with dementia* with both engendering very polarized view sets.

The well-health to ill-health transition is perhaps a clumsy way of acknowledging what is occurring especially given the regular changes that naturally take place for each person throughout their life. The focus here is driven by attitudes and the perceptual position of reimagining oneself as having to live and cope with a 'condition'. The sense here is of acknowledging 'I am a person with dementia', especially against the common rationalization of dementia being an 'old person's condition' and association with notions of senility and advancing old age. It requires a significant alteration in terms of self-perception and can cause a fair degree of anguish especially in relation to commonly associated stereotypical associations. The sense of awareness of having dementia can be an added burden to *simply* having the condition, as expressed by Terry Pratchett (2008) who was himself diagnosed with posterior cortical atrophy:

> It occurred to me that at one point it was like I had two diseases – one was Alzheimer's and the other was knowing I had Alzheimer's. There were times

> when I thought I'd have been much happier not knowing, just accepting that I'd lost brain cells and one day they'd probably grow back or whatever.

This quote expresses the impact that acknowledging one's diagnosis can have, given the powerful ways in which the term *dementia* resonates for those affected. Here 'knowing' is regarded as an additional burden to that of 'having', which illustrates the potency with which such a condition can resonate within people's lives. Indeed, a qualitative study by Lishman, Cheston and Smithson (2016) reported on the struggle in reaching acceptance:

> Just as for the child exploring a new world who needs to be able to retreat into a safe base, so people with dementia, in seeking to make sense out of the strange situation of dementia, may need to retreat back into a position where they push away or into the back of their minds thoughts of their dementia. In this sense markers of, 'warding off' or 'unwanted thoughts' equate to the 'safe base' of not knowing about their dementia to which participants can retreat as a way of reducing the emotional load. Thus, ambivalence (wanting to know, not wanting to know) regulates the pain and stress of facing the diagnosis with the need for safety and security.

It is fairly unsurprising to note the presence of these thoughts with participants wishing to retreat back to a place *before dementia* and to exist if only for a moment in a place without this spectre hovering over them. The initial period can cause extreme distress and despair with many fears for individuals concerning the road ahead. It is a path with many unknowns and anticipated struggles, fuelled by one's experiences with and observations of others with dementia, for example, parents or grandparents. The realization that one has been diagnosed with a life-changing condition can leave a person searching for answers and understanding. Kate Swaffer (2016, p.30) reacted to her diagnosis with the questions: 'Why me, why this, why now?'

She related the sensation of drowning with her familiar world disappearing and being replaced by a new uncertain one. This brief yet striking expression outlines a fascinating alternative. Here it is not so much the person changing but the world that they inhabit. This sense will clearly be reinforced through other people's changing attitudes and behaviours towards them. There may also be various modifications to their living space including complete changes in environment, for example if admitted to a care home. For many people the fears about change will be largely centred upon self. Christine Bryden (2018, p.22), herself diagnosed with dementia, commented:

> I felt oppressed by the power of the prognosis that I would gradually lose

> my sense of self, as my brain continued to atrophy; it was as if my story had become re-interpreted, re-packaged and re-presented…to conform to the objective and scientific basis of medicine.

This reinventing of self is about the emergence of a new identity through a metamorphosing process. Bryden's narrative outlines the sense of impotence present in being unable to alter or deter the powerful forces already at play, progressively wreaking their changes. John Zeisl (2010) relates Richard Taylor's message entitled 'A Plea from All the Me's I Will Be', which regards his evolving self with a sense of trepidation, desperate to hold on to something of his core being, boldly stating, 'I am still me.' The retaining of one's essential being, along with memories, is a central concern for many people with dementia. Kate Swaffer (2016) reflects upon the value for her in having her husband as her BUB (Back-Up Brain), like a USB stick to refer in the event of her own hard drive crashing, for example with assistance around memory, maths or spelling. The confidence a person has with such a process will be influenced by the degree of trust they have in others as well as the extent to which they are truly known and understood. Luft and Ingham (1955) created the Johari Window, a framework representing the different proportions of 'self' that are known entities to that person or others (Figure 4.1).

(Hidden) Known to self	(Blind) Known to others
(Open) Known to self and others	(Unknown) Known to neither self nor others

Figure 4.1 The Johari Window

One way of exploring self-awareness is by 'mapping out' the Johari Window. The name 'Johari' suggests an origin from a mystic background; however, this activity is derived from the first names of the two psychologists Joseph Luft and Harrington Ingham in 1955. The Johari Window is divided into four sections:

- the *Open* area is your open, conscious, public behaviour, which is known to you and also known to others

- the *Blind* area is where others can see things about you that you cannot see about yourself
- the *Hidden* area represents things we know about ourselves that we do not reveal to others
- the *Unknown* area includes thoughts, feelings and motives within you that are known to neither yourself nor others.

Use of this technique helps people better understand their relationship with themselves and others. The intention is to expand the open area by talking honestly about ourselves (in the form of self-disclosure) and by also listening (to the feedback from others).

ACTIVITY 4.1

Choose the person who on reflection you feel knows the most about you.

Consider examples where they:

- really understand and 'get you'
- don't really know or 'get you'.

You might have found it hard making a definite selection in Activity 4.1 as we can feel that contrasting people see different parts of us, for example parents, friends or partner, all to some degree determined by what we allow them to see. This activity highlights the significance of having around us people who could if needed act as trusted advocates, faithfully representing our wishes and needs. We might though reflect upon the old TV show *Mr and Mrs* to see how frequently people's everyday experiences, likes and dislikes were completely misinterpreted by intimate partners. This would evidently cause persons with dementia concern, for example in relation to a meal or film that was never enjoyed yet regarded by their partner and communicated to care staff as one of their favourites. Taking this further and bearing in mind Luft and Ingham's (1955) framework we can consider the following areas that a person with dementia will be concerned with:

1. what others correctly know about me
2. what others mistakenly know about me
3. what others don't know about me.

The elements in (1) will most strongly hold on to a person's core being and personhood whereas (2) and (3) will cause frustration, conflict and distress. Approaches for health carers to strengthen and appreciate core identity include the use of reminiscence and validation, which are covered in Chapter 7, 'Dementia Champions'.

As stated by MacKinlay (2012), a contemplation of life's meaning and purpose is increasingly common during the ageing process and towards the end of life. It is unsurprising that similar processes will operate for those diagnosed with dementia irrespective of age. Daly, Fahey-McCarthy and Timmins (2019) conducted a meta-synthesis considering the experiences of spirituality from the perspective of people living with a diagnosis of dementia. They regarded spirituality as a means to cope with and ascribe meaning to these events. This can be widened to conceptualize this term as representing the core of 'who we are' (Narayanasamy 2010) or, as defined by the Oxford Dictionary, as being: 'concerned with the human spirit or soul as opposed to material or physical things'.

This internal entity within a person's spiritual being is:

> Universal, deeply personal and individual; it goes beyond formal notions of ritual or religious practice to encompass the unique capacity of each individual. It is at the core and essence of who we are, that spark which permeates the entire fabric of the person and demands that we are all worthy of dignity and respect. It transcends intellectual capability, elevating the status of all humanity to that of the sacred. (McSherry 2009, cited in McSherry and Smith 2012, p.118)

Therefore, for the person diagnosed with dementia, questions posed might encompass 'Who am I?' or 'Who am I becoming?' We can also consider and incorporate what the elements are that each person might consider as making them feel truly *alive*, including experiences that stimulate and act upon senses and emotions. This can incorporate a variety of art-based approaches, also covered in Chapter 7.

A major transition brought about through one's receipt of a dementia diagnosis concerns changes in thinking, with one's mortality brought forcefully into daily thoughts and feelings. This features prominently within Thomas DeBaggio's (2002) autobiographical narrative, with his reflections regularly interrupted with ruminations around what he saw as a shortened lifespan. This mirrors what is experienced by many other people where initial thinking commonly regards a dementia diagnosis as if one were given a 'death sentence' (Bryden 2005; Young Dementia UK 2019). Activity 4.2 asks you to consider how such thought might impact upon a person.

ACTIVITY 4.2

A diagnosis of dementia can instigate fears of a shortened lifespan. Consider what feelings a person may experience in the short term in relation to:

- **a diagnosis with no cure at the present time**
- **a disease that progressively restricts/impedes a person's well-being.**

A further factor impacting upon a person's state of readiness to commence their dementia journey can relate to their anticipated losses or restrictions. For many people with young-onset dementia, a diagnosis will be given whilst they are currently engaged with a multitude of activities, occupations and responsibilities with plans already being contemplated for their future. This is all *rudely* and *cruelly* interrupted with the entrance into their lives of an experience that threatens to derail and hinder all of a person's subsequent undertakings. Becoming a *person with dementia* has the potential to resonate forcefully, with lowered expectations applied to self internally as well as from external positions. The locus of control or self-agency becomes less certain and a person's transition can be aided or hindered in relation to the support they are able to access. This is an essential aspect and as with Voyager's 'good friends' illustrates the requirement to have access to people whom one can rely upon if losing one's independence and functioning capacity. Worries around enforced dependency can heighten feelings of helplessness as well as engender fears for the potential overload caused to family members taking on a caring role. Letting go of some aspects of self-care and trusting others to assist can engender a myriad of conflicting emotions regarding one's changing role. Diana Friel McGowin (1993, p.67) recalls: 'having always been the outspoken extroverted pivotal centre of both my family and group of friends, I was now reluctantly in the non-contributing purgatory of the early diagnosed'.

This narrative outlines the fear of her position in the family shifting, presumably from the vibrancy of the centre to somewhere on the periphery, a lonelier place with lessened opportunity for feeling acknowledged. There is a core issue to consider here, namely how relationships alter in the presence of a label as powerful as that of *dementia*. Information provided by the Alzheimer's Society (2019) highlights features that will have an impact upon the family of those with young-onset dementia. They indicate that younger people with dementia are more likely to:

- be in work at the time of diagnosis
- have a partner who still works
- have dependent children
- have ageing parents who they need to care for
- be more physically fit and active
- have heavy financial commitments, such as a mortgage
- have a rarer form of dementia.

Lee, Roen and Thornton (2014) explore personal experiences of the adjustment process following a diagnosis of dementia including receiving a diagnosis and the experience of adjusting and adapting to dementia. The findings illustrated the importance, to people with Alzheimer's disease, of understanding and making sense of the diagnosis to help them deal with issues of loss and to make positive adjustments to their lives through employing specific coping strategies.

ACTIVITY 4.3

Consider what the potential impact/burden a dementia diagnosis has on Peter's life:

- regarding his self and well-being
- as a father and husband
- as a contributor to the family.

The contemplation of one's steady deterioration and loss of personal autonomy can have a detrimental impact upon a person's emotional state and ability to cope. A heightened sense of hopelessness can engender feelings of despair and pose very real risks to self, as discussed in Chapter 5. It is important to note the fluctuating positions of desperation and determination that may characterize the beginning phase of a person's dementia journey. Ways of encouraging determination can be influenced by preserving 'positive anchors' such as friends, family and peers, whilst establishing and maintaining a supportive environment that promotes an acceptance of change and retaining a person-centred outlook. This ensures that the person does not become invisible or have their dementia symptoms totally dictate their everyday interactions and relationships.

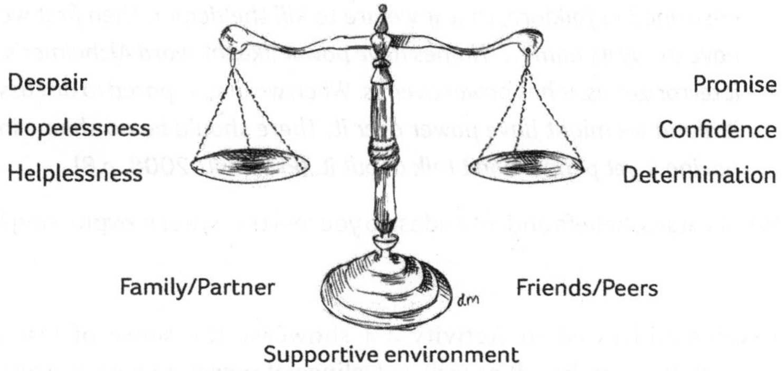

Figure 4.2 Negative and positive emotions
Source: Daisy Morris

Figure 4.2 illustrates the balancing of negative and positive emotions involved through one's contemplation of the road ahead with dementia. What this clearly illustrates is the need for elements such as family and friends and an overall environment that is supportive in order not to become totally overwhelmed and consumed by despair and hopelessness.

A 'rising to the challenge' and 'readiness to fight' was strongly verbalized by Terry Pratchett (2008) shortly after he had made his diagnosis public:

> I regarded finding I had a form of Alzheimer's as an insult, and I decided to do my best to marshal any kind of forces that I could against this wretched disease… What is needed is will and determination. The first step is to talk openly about dementia because it's a fact, well enshrined in folklore, that if we are to kill the demon, then first we have to say its name. Once we have recognised the demon, without secrecy or shame, we can find its weaknesses.

This narrative contains words and terms that convey a readiness for battle (i.e. *marshalling one's forces* and *kill the demon*) and is similarly seen in many people's responses to a cancer diagnosis (Kyngäs *et al.* 2001). We can see such an approach as a means of challenging feelings of impending mortality and seeking the vital element of *hope*. This intangible yet invaluable element provides individuals with the drive and energy to maintain their coping abilities. Terry Pratchett's determination to fight the deteriorating effects of his advancing dementia symptoms was shown in his continuation to write and publish with a series of books appearing post-diagnosis. His will to combat and deal with his dementia is highlighted in Activity 4.4.

ACTIVITY 4.4

> *The first step is to talk openly about dementia because it is a fact, well enshrined in folklore, that if we are to kill the demon then first we have to say its name... Names have power like the word Alzheimer's: it terrorizes us. It has power over us. When we are prepared to discuss it aloud we might have power over it. There should be no shame in having it yet people don't talk about it. (Pratchett 2008, p.8)*

What values, beliefs and attitudes do you feel the writer is expressing?

The issues addressed in Activity 4.4 showcase the sense of fear and uncertainty that can be felt as well as feelings of powerlessness concerning the changes taking place and one's new identity emerging. This and the other issues considered within this section illustrate the potency of elements facing the person with dementia as they commence upon their dementia journey. At the same time, a parallel process will be taking place for other family members, which will be considered within the following sections.

Partner/carer: on becoming a carer ('We are a couple with dementia')

This section is concerned with the transition that takes place for family members who adopt a caring role following a loved one's diagnosis with dementia. A commonly related aspect concerns the uncertainty as to the point at which a person actually becomes a carer, transitioning between seeing themselves more as *carer* than *partner* or *child*. The progressive and steady move towards the position of carer is outlined by Chris Carling (2012, p.5): 'Dementia, particularly Alzheimer's, is insidious, creeping up slowly, wrapping its tendrils round you, gently at first then squeezing harder.'

She related this not only to her parents having dementia but also to her own role in becoming a carer. Her expressive and metaphoric narration conjures up images of suffocation with all parties involved gradually having the life crushed out of them. This is set within her excellent autobiographical text *But Then Something Happened*, which expresses how a family can be confronted by the *spectre* of dementia that, over a series of events, brings the edifice they'd constructed tumbling down. A carer's journey, however, can contain many other elements, including positive experiences and moments of intimacy. This section will examine such issues and the thoughts and feelings individuals have at the point of contemplating taking on a caring role.

Gill's Narrative 4.2: Becoming a carer

'It is clear that Peter will need to be looked after and that responsibility will fall largely on me. Does it mean me becoming a carer? I am not at all sure I am ready to take that on at this moment in time. When I married Peter, the vows I made were just part of a ceremony and I never really contemplated what 'for better or worse' meant. Now it is "worse" and I don't know if I can manage. Part of my hesitation is about not being sure as to whether I want to. How will this affect my life? I know that may seem very selfish and uncaring given what is happening to Peter. He has no choice after all. Ashleigh is putting on a brave face, pledging to help me look after Peter. I am not so sure though if I want her to do that as she has her own family to attend to.

I don't want to give up work. The florist business is a big part of my life and I have worked so long and hard for it. I will have to speak with my partner Elizabeth about this. She knows Peter was unwell and said she will help as much as she can. She doesn't know about the dementia though and certainly can't keep covering for me indefinitely. I will also have to cut back on my leisure pursuits and membership of the leisure centre.

I have seen various things written about a "person with dementia" or "dementia patient". What about a "couple with dementia" or "family with dementia"? Is that what we are now? Are we now to be defined as a family with dementia in our midst, a lifelong mental illness without a cure?'

■ *What might Gill be feeling as she contemplates impending changes to her life and the lifestyle she values?*

You may consider completing the grid in Table 4.1 in order to explore your response to Gill's narrative.

Table 4.1 Gill's situation and outlook

Present	Future
Home situation • Relationships • Family roles Occupation • Business friendships • Financial circumstances	Home situation • Relationships • Family roles Occupation • Business friendships • Financial circumstances

cont.

Present	Future
Gill's present outlook...	Gill's future outlook... ....

Gill's narrative is a very striking example of the multitude of emotions and concerns faced by partners at the start of the dementia journey. Whilst a caring role might be shared by a number of individuals including healthcare professionals, there will certainly be a sense of responsibility and expectation upon partners or maybe grown-up children where there is no partner or where the partner is unable for various reasons such as ill-health to take on this role. Gill expresses trepidation and fear at a number of aspects, questioning her ability to take on a caring role. The transition and changes will impact upon her life in important ways involving having to give up or restrict things important to her, including her engagement with the florist business. Essentially, the contemplation of changes that lie ahead for the prospective carer can involve:

- What does it mean being a couple with dementia?
- How will this impact upon me and change my life?
- How will this impact upon and change us as a family?

ACTIVITY 4.5

Consider all of the varied aspects of Gill's life that she is having to consider giving up or restricting.

- **What do you think will be the biggest difficulty for her?**
- **How might these issues impact upon her well-being?**

The changes for Gill as described in her narrative involve having to contemplate giving up occupations and activities that are important to her and help define who she is. She is also faced with redefining her role in relation to Peter. Activity 4.5 asked you to consider what Gill might be faced with losing. Such a contemplation will evidently resonate powerfully upon those concerned and we can also question to what extent this might affect a person's resolve to embark on their caring responsibilities. This will clearly also result in changes within their resultant relationship with their dependant partner. Living with a serious condition such as dementia means having to contemplate changes, with dependency issues becoming more apparent. In many cases it will require a family to reorganize and redistribute roles including the taking on of caring responsibilities. A person's feelings about taking on a caring role will differ according to who the individual concerned is and their relationship to the person requiring help. It might entail familial care and support being provided by a partner, child, or more strikingly perhaps, by a parent. We can also consider care being provided by other family members, friends and neighbours. A caring role towards the person concerned may already exist or there might be a situation with roles needing to be reversed. In the case of Gill where she and Peter were relatively independent and reciprocal care was provided, the commencement of a caring role will have powerful implications upon Gill's employment and leisure activities. Indeed, Gill's narrative illustrates her doubts about taking on a caring role in relation to the perceived physical and emotional demands involved. Thoughts about becoming the principal carer for her husband are likely to impact upon their relationship together, especially when, for example, considering having to assist with Peter's intimate personal care. The adoption of a caring role for one's partner will engender varying degrees of willingness or reluctance. For some, there may be an acknowledgement that this is a role or duty expected from one's partner and the sense that he or she would do the same for me. For others, the caring role may be adopted mainly on account of there being a lack of alternative options. It might also be taken on more rigorously in order to protect other family members, especially children, which was seen in Gill's narrative concerning her daughter Ashleigh.

As indicated previously, an aspect that might be hard to determine concerns the point at which a person actively considers themselves to be a carer. For some it might be a rapid transformation if, for example, a person's cognitive decline occurs very quickly, whilst for others the role might appear to progress very gradually with no clear delineation between positions of partner (non-carer) and carer: 'It is a role that can come unexpectedly out of a crisis; it is a role that can creep up on you' (Department of Health and Social Care 2010).

The internet site Healthtalk (2019) features interviews with family carers of individuals with dementia. One narrative outlines how the role of carer was taken on:

> I have to do his personal care now. I have to wash and he dresses himself still, very slowly and sometimes I have to help him, but I think you gradually

> slot into this role of carer. If somebody came along and said to you 'You're going to be a carer in two years' time, a full time carer', you'd say 'No way.' But because it sneaks up on you…you take it on.

This highlights the insidious nature of a role that develops progressively over time. It is telling, however, that the narrator here expresses the feeling that they would have declined such a role if not being caught unaware. Despite such declarations, the point of actually being faced with a family member's plight will create a huge dilemma and can involve a balancing of caring against existing work and family responsibilities. Indeed, the commencement of carers' journeys are commonly marked by what Griffin *et al.*'s (2016) study noted as feelings of *bewilderment* where subsequent decisions and actions can be carried out as if in a daze. A study by Dunham and Dietz (2003) found women caregivers expressing worries that they would not be able to give their family members the care they deserved because of the multiple demands placed on them. A number of women actively negotiated working conditions to achieve greater flexibility, although this would in turn have financial consequences. Work can also provide respite and a bolster to one's self-esteem as well as fulfilling a core social need. In spite of the importance of work to them, these women paid costs for balancing both roles.

The term 'carer' makes an assumption that a person has chosen to take on this role and adopt a way of life where they will witnesses changes in their partner, relative or friend that can redefine existing and established relationships. A consequence of becoming a carer is a growing sense of isolation and feeling marginalized, which may engender thoughts around how and why they have become a carer, where *choice* or *circumstances* can influence how they view their new role. Interventions in dementia care evidently need to include both halves of the 'care-giving dyad' (Charlesworth 2001), which in this instance concerns supporting Gill and Peter's present and future relationship. Harris and Keady (2009) argue that maintaining and sustaining a sense of self-identity and independence is a critical feature of adulthood but for people diagnosed with dementia this can become a daunting and complex challenge. Some individuals with early-onset dementia, during their mid-life, may be forced to face tasks of later life too soon and potentially prior to the successful resolution of any outstanding crises from their mid-life.

We can consider individuals such as Chris Carling or the TV presenter Fiona Phillips who returned to a caring role when faced with a second parent being diagnosed with dementia. In such cases the individual is cognisant of the fact that they will become a carer again and with full understanding of what this entails yet still engages in this role. The fact that caring responsibilities are taken on despite having an awareness of how totally consuming and distressing it can be shows how potent family ties are. Indeed, as reflected by Gerrard (2019, p.118), it is a role that has the capacity to be many things such as: 'exhausting, farcical, revelatory, horrifying, enriching, tragic'.

She further comments upon the limitations for reciprocity and Professor Sally Gadow's reflection upon the caring role as 'a process of entering another's vulnerability and brokenness and breaking oneself' (Gerrard 2019, p.119). This powerful statement including the notion 'breaking oneself' illustrates the impact upon carers and their preparation and readiness for the emotional rollercoaster which lies ahead.

Part of the difficulty for carers involves the apparent limitation of alternatives, feeling that to not take on the caring role, however ill-equipped they might feel to cope, would mean abandoning their family member. This is illustrated by a carer interviewed for the Healthtalk (2019) site who, after visiting a care centre and being displeased about how it was run, made the decision to look after his partner: 'If she were gonna be looked after anywhere it was gonna be here where she could have whatever she needed and somebody to look after her interests, because there's so many people whose interests are not looked after.'

This starkly highlights the dilemma facing many carers with the feeling that others would not care as diligently for their loved one, which strengthens one's resolve to take on their care despite the personal costs that may be involved. This points to a feeling of being trapped, an experience reflected within the following narrative. Andrea Gillies (2009, p.31) writes very openly in her book *Keeper* about her experience of caring for her mother-in-law with dementia in a remote region of Scotland:

> Taking on Nancy's care, full time, seven days, 24 hours, has been… I wish I could find a better word than shock. It's been a shock. The thesaurus offers 'trauma' but that isn't remotely it. It hasn't been a 'blow' or an 'upset', a 'bombshell' or a 'jolt'. It's more the kind of experience that leaves you staring into space open-mouthed. How on earth did I get here, you think. And how am I going to extricate myself… I have a new role, a new identity.

This narrative illustrates all too plainly how trapped she felt within what was recounted as the relentless nature of her caring role. Her expressive text takes us inside the 'shock' and examines what it felt like for her with the daily challenges she had to face. The statement about having 'a new identity' hints at a reinvention of self and acknowledgement of one's emerging caring role. It in a sense outlines how a person is subsequently to be defined. Reviews and feedback concerning this text were overwhelmingly positive and it is illuminating reading the responses at Amazon's website and noting the number of fellow carers who express a strong connection and feeling of engagement with Gillies' text.

> Helpful to anyone with a family member suffering with dementia. This isn't, inevitably, a happy-ever-after story, but one which should help anyone feel that they are not alone if they find themselves, often painfully and scarily, in a similar situation.
>
> My husband has Alzheimers, and I wondered if I would be able to face reading this book…it explains what is happening to my husband and makes it easier for me to be understanding and patient in daily living when I know which parts of the brain are ceasing to function and the effect that has.

The examples cited above show how important it is to talk about and share experiences of caring. This promotes further dialogue and conversations around experiences and difficulties that individuals might be struggling with. There is a sense of *permission-giving* for sharing thoughts and feelings including those at the more desperate and hopeless end of the spectrum. The feedback shows the value in feeling connected with others and acknowledging that there are others who 'get it' in terms of properly having an awareness of what individuals are going through. As with Yalom's (2005) curative concept of *universality*, this promotes the feeling that one is not alone.

We are a couple with dementia

The presence of an illness or condition within a family member can result in relationships being redefined and newly understood. Being a *couple with dementia* can feel very different from simply seeing selves as a couple. The presence of the condition or term attached to the preposition 'with' can take on a predominance above that of the people it is related to. As the term 'dementia' is prone to be regarded with such pessimism and uncertainty, the attachment of this term to that of 'couple' will in many people's minds threaten and undermine the foundations of that partnership. Robinson, Clare and Evans' (2005) findings suggest that couples who receive a diagnosis of dementia may be supported by helping them to create a joint construction that enables them to make sense of their situation, find ways of adjusting to the changes experienced in their roles and identity and manage the losses they face in the early stages of dementia.

The need for this is supported by Ducharme *et al.* (2011) who report on the results of a pro-active psycho-educational programme in aiding the transition to a caregiver role following the diagnosis of Alzheimer's disease in a relative. Caregivers involved perceived themselves to be better prepared to provide care, were better able to plan for the future care needs of their relative, had better knowledge of available services and employed further coping strategies. This highlights the core importance of healthcare professionals aiding family members in adjusting to their new roles, something that clearly extends to wider family members.

ACTIVITY 4.6

What would it mean for you if you became a carer?

What could get in the way for you?

EXERCISE: CHANGING RELATIONSHIPS ON BECOMING A CARER

This exercise asks the reader to explore their understanding of the ways relationships can change when becoming a carer. (See Chapter 8.)

Participants in Adams' (2006) study were asked to describe the earliest changes in the parent or spouse and the changes to their everyday lives and in their relationships brought by cognitive impairment. These family members reported taking on many new responsibilities, especially decision-making and supervision. The majority of participants reported experiencing frustration, resentment, grief and relational deprivation, along with increased protectiveness and tenderness towards the person with dementia. It was also notable that a large number of participants reported ambivalence about seeking or accepting help from others, striving to maintain the status quo for as long as possible. If we try and unpick the meaning of this, we might note the number of contributory factors including the fact that to accept help means acknowledging that there is a problem, something that families may find very difficult to do. There is also the issue of seeking help and not really knowing what this entails or its implications.

Robinson *et al.* (2011) found that the key challenges for family carers related to the process of becoming the main decision-maker and adjusting to increased responsibility. This indicates raised levels of stress and pressure for those concerned, and during the initial period of caring family members can potentially neglect their own needs. Caring for partners and family members will engender a number of decisions that in many instances are made alone.

Shim *et al.* (2013) express that whilst dementia caregiving can be burdensome and challenging for spousal caregivers, it can also be an opportunity for growth and transcendence. This is a valid point and one worth noting, as although there are many feared consequences for couples connected with the dementia experience there can be some very strong positives including people feeling more engaged and closer to each other. Diana Melly, struggling for years with feelings of bitterness over her husband George's infidelities and errant behaviour, noted:

> At the end, it was really just the two of us and we became good friends again. In some ways, it was the same as it had been at the beginning of our relationship. Everything seemed to come full circle and it was such a natural progression. (*Evening Standard* 2007)

This was also reflected in the BBC documentary *George Melly's Last Stand* (2007) where the tenderness and closeness between the couple was very clearly shown.

A dilemma expressed within Gill's narrative concerns the contemplation of having to stop work with her caring role expected to steadily increase. The ability to retain a work role can be reliant upon available support mechanisms and resources. Rachael Dixey (2010) was younger than her partner with dementia and continued to work through setting up a rota of paid helpers and friends to assist. This situation was partially driven by financial reasons, but also the feeling that it wouldn't be good for their partnership to be together all of the time given the difficulties faced. For some carers, such support is unavailable and retaining a working role is only done by adjusting one's hours. Michael Fassio (2009) recounts becoming the main carer for his mother Renza and being advised by colleagues to reduce his hours and not to give up work completely. This, he reflected, provided him with a moderate stream of income as well as a vital link to the outside world. The external contact provided him with a lifeline, especially given his gradually constricting social life. It shows some of the crucial needs being met through employment, including a sense of purpose, enhanced self-esteem and added financial security. Even reduced working hours, though, can eventually become unsustainable as experienced by Duncan (2010) who finally stopped work altogether when the stress of concurrently caring for her mother became too much. There is a clear conflict and tension here for individuals desperately trying to hold on to a work role and the lifeline provided yet at the same time feeling unable to cope with the pressure of their caring role, which can include multiple dependants. An interviewee on the Healthtalk (2019) site expressed:

> I just wish I could be signed off work for a month, I don't know what's going to happen next week, especially because work has put an added responsibility on me now...something will have to give. So yes it's difficult. I can manage my mother and my daughter and my granddaughter I think, if I could just get rid of work, yes it is difficult. Yes, there have been times when I've been breaking up.

This illustrates the lability of this narrator's thoughts, struggling to find an appropriate solution but uncertain as to what to do. It is decisions such as this and those addressed above that mark the carer's experience. The sheer difficulty in knowing what choices to make and how to proceed will no doubt feel overwhelming and goes some way towards acknowledging the sense of *bewilderment* noted by Griffin *et al.*'s (2016) study of carers at the start of their dementia journey.

In 2010 the government proposed a selection of actions to support carers and those they were looking after. Their strategy included:

- supporting those with caring responsibilities to identify themselves as carers at an early stage, recognizing the value of their contribution and involving them from the outset both in designing local care provision and in planning individual care packages
- enabling those with caring responsibilities to fulfil their educational and employment potential
- offering personalized support for carers and those they support, enabling them to engage fully in family and community life.

ACTIVITY 4.7

What carers' strategies exist where you live?

How do your local health and social care organizations promote their carer intentions?

When were their first publications and how often are they reviewed?

Reflecting upon the picture worldwide, Glasby and Thomas (2019) highlight the estimated number of dementia carers as:

- Australia: 291,163 (413,106 people with dementia)
- UK: 700,000 (850,000 people with dementia)
- US: 16.1 million (5.8 million people with dementia).

Some of the related available support includes:

- Australia: free counselling services offered by Dementia Australia and the Carer Gateway Counselling Service
- UK: Admiral Nurses Carer Information and Support Programme (Alzheimer's Society)
- US: in-person support groups (Alzheimer's Association); specialist guidance from the National Alliance for Caregiving.

Amongst the support noted above we can consider the UK-based service available from professional carers through the Admiral Nursing service. John Suchet (2010) reflects upon some of the ways in which his allocated nurse has helped him through having space to express and explore his feelings, understanding his and his wife Bonnie's behaviour, and by acknowledging that it can be normal to lose his temper and have an 'off day'. This service is only available in certain geographical locations within the UK.

Children/family members: role transitions ('We are a family with dementia')

For family members, the period following diagnosis can be characterized by much uncertainty and an adjustment of roles. Gelman and Rhames (2016) conduced 12 in-depth interviews with children and well parents in families with a parent with young-onset dementia on the experience and needs of children having a parent with this diagnosis. Children reported disruption in many aspects of their lives in relation to their developmental trajectory, emotional and psychological development, familial and broader social relationships, and financial stability. We can also consider tension amongst family members involving the distribution and uptake of caring responsibilities. Blandin and Pepin (2017) posit that it is 'normal' for parent–child relationships to go through a challenging period during adolescence and for those whose parent develops dementia at this time, resolution and restoration of amicability may not be possible, causing further and potentially lasting distress. This section examines these issues with a specific focus upon younger family members, especially children and adolescents. As healthcare providers predominantly tailor their care packages towards the person diagnosed with dementia followed by attention upon primary family caregivers, others such as children in the family are prone to being overlooked. The powerful changes taking place within the family will cause much distress, confusion and anguish amongst younger family members who can be dissuaded from talking about and expressing their feelings because of the protectiveness extended by others. The issues facing them and what this means in terms of their lived experience are addressed within this section.

Ashleigh's Narrative 4.3: Feeling impotent

'When I think of the future I feel very worried for my parents. It is just heart-breaking seeing the changes in Dad, someone who has always been so proudly independent and capable. Mum seems exhausted all the time now and I wish I knew how to help her more. Things will only get harder for her and I have no idea how she is going to cope. I must admit I find it hard enough caring for my daughter Hannah and am struggling to find opportunities to help out more. I do visit whenever I can and assist with the house and shopping. My husband Chris is very supportive although I am scared that our relationship will suffer because of the limited time we get to spend together with just the two of us. I wish Matt would lend a hand although he just seems totally uninterested and removed from what is going on. He says he has his studies to attend to but don't we all have other things to do? Tom is too young to really get involved and shouldn't be "babysitting" his own father. I mean how crazy would that be? Can I really divide myself up and properly attend to everyone's needs?'

Matt's Narrative 4.4: Feeling detached

'Dad is getting worse and I don't know how to respond. When he and Mum visited recently I just felt so awkward and uncomfortable. They met briefly with my friends and I was simply willing Dad to keep quiet lest anyone discover his dementia. I haven't told anyone here at uni – that would I suppose make it feel more real. I resist phoning home or visiting as much as possible and when I do I keep the conversation brief and on lighter topics in order to not have to face what is going on. I am very stressed with my exams and endless number of essays, which aren't really going very well. I simply can't concentrate on my work.'

Tom's Narrative 4.5: Feeling bewildered

'I wish somebody would tell me what is happening as I always seem to be the last person to find out anything. The situation at home is going to get worse, I can see that. Mum has asked me to stay in on occasions whilst she goes shopping. Essentially that means I am to babysit Dad. I mean how mixed up is that? He is only going to get more forgetful, which will mean an increase in having to be looked after. I want to help but it all feels too painful as every new problem reminds me that I am losing my Dad.'

- *If you were one of the Lawrence children, what could you be feeling at the present time?*
- *Select one of the children and in that role ask yourself: what support could I realistically offer Mum and Dad?*

Ashleigh's narrative provides a stark expression of the predicament faced by younger family members trying to come to terms with what is happening to their family whilst simultaneously attempting to juggle other existing responsibilities. The introduction of further caring responsibilities is a concern and viewed with trepidation given the impact that this is likely to have. It can be compared with the anguished and frantic position faced by plate spinners who are already struggling to keep them rotating whilst witnessing additional crockery being added. Observing the progressive exhaustion and stress of family carers will cause significant distress and engender a desire to help and protect them. In Ashleigh's case she has competing responsibilities with her work and family. She expresses her worry about having limited time to spend with her young daughter Hannah and husband Chris, but perhaps her unexpressed fear concerns the potential absence for her of 'me time'. A core element here will be exhaustion with insufficient time for rest and restoration. Given the often protracted nature of dementia, family caregivers may face particular difficulties. Leggett *et al.* (2018) found that many dementia caregivers report sleep disturbances, and those who find caregiving more upsetting are more likely to experience disrupted sleep.

The tension between siblings is shown in Ashleigh's narrative with a glimmer of resentment creeping out towards Matt, her largely absent sibling. Whilst there is some rationalization and understanding of his situation, feelings of resentment and grievance can grow and develop between family members, especially if one's personal burdens become intolerable. A stark illustration of the need for family members to feel that others are sharing responsibility is contained in Michael Ignatieff's (1993) excellent fictional narrative *Scar Tissue*. In this text the narrator requests that his brother accompanies him and their mother to a care home facility for the purpose of dividing the associated feelings of guilt. Historically, adult child caregivers may experience more family conflict than partner caregivers, as they often have to negotiate the caregiving role with siblings (Strawbridge and Wallhagen 1991). If we take the time to consider what Matt, the absent sibling, might be experiencing, his apparent lack of interest and separateness could be better understood. His above narrative provides us with plenty of clues. Here we see his discomfort and uncertainty as to how to respond to other family members and his attempt to cope through avoidance and distancing himself. It is clearly not an effective approach and the strain is evidently showing. Related to this, a participant in Hall and Sikes's (2017) study around children of parents with dementia reflected upon his coping through 'detachment':

> Recently I've said to my Dad when I've really not been coping 'I'm beyond caring, I just wanna turn my back and walk away' ... Which is obviously an awful thing to say but, there's a bit of logic to it because I don't really see what the advantage is in putting myself through it all the time when I could quite easily detach myself completely, and in a way, I already have part detached that allows me to get on with my life.

What we see here is the need for support and opportunities for those in this position to begin to express themselves and work through their feelings. As well as being helpful for the individual concerned it would also help them with the offering of support for other family members.

Ashleigh's concerns about Tom show the conflict with wanting to protect younger and more vulnerable family members. Such a concern is understandable given the frequently cited lack of support received by young carers. The Alzheimer's Society (2016) present Charlotte's story, who between the ages of 8 and 16 helped to care for three of her grandparents with dementia. The strain of this role impacted significantly upon her health and well-being. She felt exhausted most of the time, isolated herself from peers and struggled with her schooling. She referred to herself as a 'hidden carer', with healthcare professionals, family and friends unaware as to what she was going through. Similarly, Clare Brien, who featured in the 2014 Channel 4 documentary *Britain's Youngest Carers*, took on a caring role for her father (and mother with physical health needs) at the age of ten following his development of vascular dementia following a stroke. She related the anguish and distress felt at seeing someone so close to her suddenly rendered so vulnerable and helpless. School and college work as well as friends were routinely put to the side whilst she carried out her caring role. This all reflects what Tom, Matt and Ashleigh might be experiencing, each with their own struggle and experienced difficulty yet feeling alone with it. It is important to note that young people and children can invest in the caring dynamic even if not regarded as *carers*. Care can be engaged in through means other than providing practical support and includes engagement emotionally and psychologically. It is key that health carers recognize this and extend their involvement to encompass the whole family. This is reflected by Nichols *et al.* (2013) who identified opportunities for professionals to assist young carers in overcoming stigma and the challenge of balancing childhood and adolescent development within this context.

The protectiveness towards younger family members can be such that they are kept ignorant of what is occurring and without opportunities or *permission* to share and express their feelings. Helen Beaumont (2009) had two young children (aged three and four) to consider when her husband Clive was diagnosed with dementia at the age of 45. She stressed the need to desist in protecting children by keeping them unaware of what is going on. She also advocated the importance of scheduling time in a family's routine when the children can talk, together and individually, with the parent who does not have dementia. Acknowledging the changes and worries that young family members can have can certainly be alleviated through talking as well as accessing resources for awareness-raising.

There are some interesting resources aimed at promoting awareness in children about a family member's dementia. Russell and Johnston's (2017) *Grandma Forgets* is a book that is essentially about holding memories for those who are no longer able to. It stresses the value in recalling what is important about a person with dementia and our shared time with them. This reflects the importance of reminiscence, an approach strongly advocated within the TV documentary *Dementiaville* where Dr David Sheard introduced approaches for families to continue sharing activities and experiences that have a strong sense of resonance for them. Another resource, Prior and Drummond's (2018) *Grandma and Me: A Kid's Guide for Alzheimer's and Dementia*, is cited as a book that explains what is happening to those with dementia. It is narrated from a child's perspective and illustrates the need for children to understand and better cope with their feelings. It also importantly notes that a person with dementia's behaviour is not directed at or caused by them. This book essentially looks at how to maintain a relationship and how to engage in what is termed 'meet me where I am care'. Amazon product feedback illustrates how helpful families have found it in explaining dynamics to young children. There are a number of similar books about a grandparent with dementia but what are perhaps absent are books for children centring upon a *parent* with dementia. This is a point made by Kate Swaffer (2016) with thoughts about her children's understanding and acknowledgement of her dementia diagnosis.

A significant difficulty includes the redefining of identity not just of individuals but also of couples and families. This includes the realization and acknowledgement of 'we are a family with dementia', which can be resisted by members unwilling to accept this on account of the negatively associated elements. Each person is likely to have their own individual conception about what the condition of dementia encapsulates and its implications:

- Gill may ask herself whether she is willing, prepared or able to become Peter's carer.
- Ashleigh may ask herself how she can support her dad with his deteriorating condition, her mum with her caring role, her siblings with their distress as well as spending quality time with her husband and young daughter.
- Matt may ask himself whether he is prepared to accept what is happening within his family and whether it feels easier to keep his distance.
- Tom may ask himself what he can do to help in his limited capacity as well as to consider who might be there for him.

When a person is caring for someone with dementia there can be negative consequences for that carer; this phenomenon has become known as caregiver burden. A World Health Organization's report (2017) outlined a global action plan emphasizing the need to prepare for and try to prevent some of the personal and financial burden of dementia. This action plan on the public health response to dementia, 2017 to 2025, aims to improve the lives of people with dementia, their carers and families, while decreasing the possible impact of dementia on communities and countries. In support of a world vision where dementia is prevented and people with dementia and their carers are able to receive the care and support they need to live a life with meaning and dignity, they highlight areas for the action plan:

- dementia as a public health priority
- dementia awareness and friendliness
- risk reduction

- diagnosis, treatment, care and support
- support for dementia carers
- strengthening information systems for dementia
- research and innovation.

In 2018, Alzheimer's Disease International (ADI), a global federation of Alzheimer's disease associations, published *From Plan to Impact*, highlighting that not enough progress had been made and that governments worldwide need to make dementia a higher priority and must take action quickly to prevent the burden of dementia becoming overwhelming. The ADI intends to publish a new edition every year on the progress achieved; however, this first publication is not that encouraging.

Because a diagnosis of young-onset dementia commonly occurs in a person's forties and fifties there will likely be an impact upon individuals' abilities to meet familial responsibilities. Whilst memory loss may be a primary feature of young-onset dementia, initial symptoms can include uncharacteristic behavioural changes. A diagnosis should be seen as unique to the person even though the person shares a *dementia name* with many others. For example, vascular dementia, dementia with Lewy bodies, young-onset Alzheimer's, posterior cortical atrophy and dementias associated with Huntington's, Parkinson's disease, and alcoholism (Korsakoff's syndrome). Not wishing to generalize and thereby lose sight of the person within, their observable signs and symptoms might include a variety of behaviours that cause difficulties for family members. These might include aggression, social withdrawal, disinhibitions, diminished lack of empathy and hyper-sexuality. There may also be difficulties with communication, judgement-making and experienced hallucinations. Such features will clearly have a strong effect upon children and adolescents causing them much confusion and distress. We have an example in the documentary *The Trouble with Dad* (2017) with a young girl confronted on an increasing basis by abuse and swearing from her father with Pick's disease. Within the same programme we witness David Baddiel and his brother also being verbally abused by their father, who has been diagnosed with the same condition. Whereas they appear to be fairly well prepared to accept that this behaviour is driven by an organic condition, such experiences will clearly cause significant conflict within a child's emotional understanding.

Tom's struggle when spending time with his father was in part generated by being confronted with what was being lost. Each activity engaged in stimulated recollections of shared time together, which, whilst helping to hold on to their relationship, also evoked feelings of pain. His narrative also outlined his difficulty in accepting his role reversal as well as the distress in watching his father's decline. Allen, Oyebode and Allen (2009) investigated the impact of having a father with young-onset dementia on young people's well-being. The study interviewed 12 children aged 13 to 23 years about their experiences. The main themes reported included the stress of difficult behaviours associated with dementia, along with the need to reconfigure family relationships as a result. Findings also highlighted the physical and emotional strain of providing care. Svanberg, Stott and Spector (2010) conducted in-depth interviews with 12 children aged between 11 and 17 years in the UK who had a parent diagnosed with young-onset dementia. A range of feelings and experiences were expressed describing the disruption in family life of having a parent diagnosed and the challenges of acknowledging the loss of a parent as role model and caretaker, subsequently having to develop a new type of relationship with them. These studies illustrate the disruption caused to a family's identity and the resultant changes in role and structure required.

A further issue concerns that of role transition between parent and child. This is shown by Johannessen, Engedal and Thorsen's (2015) study involving in-depth interviews with 14 young Norwegian adults aged between 18 and 30 years who had grown up with a parent with young-onset dementia. The themes identified included 'my parent is sliding away', 'emotional chaos', 'becoming a parent to my parent' and 'battle'. This daunting role reversal of a child adopting the parental role was shown in Allen *et al.*'s (2009) study as strongly impacting upon young people with the stress of taking on a father's role as protector to the family. These studies illustrate some very powerful changes in family structure and roles. For a young person required to *parent* their own parent we can question how it might impact upon their subsequent relationship and how imbalanced it is likely to feel. The dynamics here will become more complex where for example a clash of cultures is experienced. Hamad *et al.* (2017) outline the variability that exists within the dementia experience of individuals, families and social groups from various cultures. They note the potential familial tensions and challenges where there may exist an intergenerational and cultural clash between family members, for example between Western and Eastern philosophies and beliefs around health and illness.

Research by Hall and Sikes (2017) on young people whose parents have dementia highlighted some striking issues with participants talking about *cancer envy*. This focused upon parents living with cancer still being able to communicate, advise and provide educational and financial support, as well as helping to resolve relationship problems, which are common to adolescence. Data from the 22 participants, the majority aged between

18 and 24 years, described a parent diagnosed with young-onset dementia as being different from how they formerly were and periodically behaving in unpleasant, difficult and embarrassing ways. This was at a time in their lives when they were already experiencing stress from the educational work and exams they were concurrently engaged in. Matt's narrative is illustrative of this dynamic acting in denial and beginning to struggle with his studies.

This section has shown the struggle faced by young people and children when having dementia as an entity to consider within their family. Whether they see themselves as having a caring role or not they still have distinct needs for support and recognition as to what they are experiencing and feeling, something for healthcare professionals to take heed of when working with individuals with dementia.

How true could this be today?

The theme of 'How true could this be today?' asks you to consider reframing an observation from the past. This commentary had an influence in informing thinking at that time whilst also determining opinions of the day. A number of questions will encourage you to consider its relevance in the here and now, such as: have national opinions changed or not? Do you agree or not with these comments? What has influenced your attitudes?

Background information: in 1950s America a number of psychologists argued that humans are motivated by the uniquely human need to expand their frontiers and to realize as much of their potential as possible. Maslow (1954) arranged human needs in a hierarchical order where basic needs have to be satisfied as a basis to strive to meet higher needs (physiological – safety – love and belonging – esteem – self-actualization). He called striving to achieve one's personal potential 'self-actualization'. Furthermore Maslow described esteem needs as contributing to the 'feeling of self-confidence, worth, strength, capacity, and adequacy, of being useful and necessary in the world' (1970, p.45).

- Do you agree or not with these observations from the 1950s?
- Do you agree or not with the comments made about esteem needs in the 1970s?
- Can you identify what your esteem needs could be (for example, being treated in a dignified manner, being respected, feeling useful and productive)?
- What do you think Peter's esteem needs could be as he commences his dementia journey?

Concluding thoughts

This chapter has addressed the nature of role transitions with the condition *dementia* gaining a foothold within a family's perceptual frameworks. This includes the recognition and acceptance of being a person, couple and family *with dementia*. It involves a significant shift in orientation and structure with tensions created in relationships. This realization brings with it fears for the future and uncertainty around the impact upon the family unit. Part of this concerns present and impending losses coupled with a strong sense of uncertainty and helplessness. A balancing act is needed with feelings such as despair, fear and hopelessness contrasted by a surrounding environment of support. As shown through the narratives and themes explored there are clear needs for all parties. The particular difficulties faced through the dementia journey are examined within the following chapter.

PERSONAL LEARNING

What was your past knowledge and understanding, what new learning have you achieved and how could this inform your future personal and/or professional interventions?

As a 'family member', my new learning includes ....

....

On reading the first-person narratives, my new learning includes

....

INTERVENTIONS

Be mindful that whatever comments are offered should be realistic, achievable and person centred. Also, that the feelings conveyed and observations made reinforce the 'dementia journey' for the individual and significant other people in their life.

The types of interventions could include ....

....

References

Adams, K. (2006). 'The transition to caregiving: the experience of family members embarking on the dementia caregiving career.' *Journal of Gerontological Social Work 47* (3–4), 3–29.

Allen, J., Oyebode, J. and Allen, J. (2009). 'Having a father with young onset dementia: the impact on well-being of young people.' *Dementia 8* (4), 455–480.

Alzheimer's Association (n.d.). *Support Groups*. Accessed on 31/1/20 at www.alz.org/events/event_search?etid=2&cid=0.

Alzheimer's Disease International (2018). *From Plan to Impact. Progress Towards Targets of the Global Action Plan on Dementia*. London: Alzheimer's Disease International.

Alzheimer's Society (n.d.). *Carer Information and Support Programme*. Accessed on 31/1/20 at www.alzheimers.org.uk/about-us/our-dementia-programmes/carer-information-support-programme.

Alzheimer's Society (2016). *A Teenager Speaks Out About the Strain of Being a Young Carer*. Accessed on 15/6/19 at www.alzheimers.org.uk/get-support/publications-and-factsheets/dementia-together-magazine/young-carer.

Alzheimer's Society (2019). *Particular Issues Faced by Young People with Dementia*. Accessed on 6/1/20 at www.alzheimers.org.uk/about-dementia/types-dementia/particular-issues-faced-younger-people-dementia#content-start.

Beaumont, H. (2009). *Losing Clive to Younger Onset Dementia*. London: Jessica Kingsley Publishers.

Blandin, K. and Pepin, R. (2017). 'Dementia grief: a theoretical model of a unique grief experience.' *Dementia 16* (1), 67–78.

Bryden, C. (2005). *Dancing with Dementia*. London: Jessica Kingsley Publishers.

Bryden, C. (2018). *Will I Still Be Me? Finding a Continuing Sense of Self in the Lived Experience of Dementia*. London: Jessica Kingsley Publishers.

Carer Gateway Counselling Service (n.d.). *Welcome to the Carer Gateway Counselling Service*. Accessed on 31/1/20 at https://counselling.carergateway.gov.au/s.

Carling, C. (2012). *But Then Something Happened*. Cambridge: Golden Books.

Charlesworth, G. (2001). 'Reviewing psychosocial interventions for family carers of people with dementia.' *Aging and Mental Health* 5, 104–106.

Daly, L., Fahey-McCarthy, E. and Timmins, F. (2019). 'The experience of spirituality from the perspective of people living with dementia: a systematic review and meta-synthesis.' *Dementia 8* (2), 448–470.

DeBaggio, T. (2002). *Losing My Mind: An Intimate Look at Alzheimer's*. New York: The Free Press.

Dementia Australia (n.d.). *Counselling*. Accessed on 31/1/20 at www.dementia.org.au/support/services-and-programs/services-and-programs/counselling-qld.

Department of Health and Social Care (2010). *Recognised, Valued and Supported: Next Steps for the Carers Strategy*. London: HMSO.

Dixey, R. (2010). 'Walking on thin ice.' In L. Whitman (ed.) *Telling Tales About Dementia: Experiences of Caring*. London: Jessica Kingsley Publishers.

Ducharme, F., Levesque, L., Lachance, L., Kergoat, M., Legault, A., Beaudet, M. and Zarit, S. (2011). 'Learning to become a family caregiver: efficacy of an intervention program for caregivers following diagnosis of dementia in a relative.' *Gerontologist 51* (4), 484–489.

Duncan, M. (2010). 'This has gone beyond my mother.' In L. Whitman (ed.) *Telling Tales About Dementia: Experiences of Caring*. London: Jessica Kingsley Publishers.

Dunham, C. and Dietz, B. (2003). 'If I'm not allowed to put my family first: challenges experienced by women who are caregiving for family members with dementia.' *Journal of Women and Aging 15* (1), 55–69.

Evening Standard (2007). 'I Wanted to Kill George, Says Wife Diana Melly.' 13 July. Accessed on 29/3/20 at www.standard.co.uk/showbiz/i-wanted-to-kill-george-says-wife-diana-melly-6597702.html.

Fassio, M. (2009). *Dementia and Mum. Who Really Cares?* London: Kew Bridge Press.

Friel McGowin, D. (1993). *Living in the Labyrinth: A Personal Journey through the Maze of Alzheimer's*. New York: Delacorte Press.

Gelman, C. and Rhames, K. (2016). 'In their own words: the experience and needs of children in younger-onset Alzheimer's disease and other dementias families.' *Dementia 17* (3), 263–265.

Gerrard, N. (2019). *What Dementia Teaches Us About Love*. London: Allen Lane.

Gillies, A. (2009). *Keeper: Living with Nancy*. London: Short Books.

Griffin, J., Oyebode, J.R. and Allen, J. (2016). 'Living with a diagnosis of behavioural-variant frontotemporal dementia: the person's experience.' *Dementia 15* (6), 1622–1642.

Glasby, J. and Thomas, S. (2019). *Understanding and Responding to the Needs of the Carers of People with Dementia in the UK, the US and Beyond.* Accessed on 31/1/20 at https://lx.iriss.org.uk/sites/default/files/carers-of-people-with-dementia.pdf.

Hall, M. and Sikes, P. (2017). '"It would be easier if she'd died": young people with parents with dementia articulating inadmissible stories.' *Qualitative Health Research 27* (8), 1203–1214.

Hamad, E., AlHadi, A., Lee, C., Savundranayagam, M., Holmes, J., Kinsella, E. and Johnson, A. (2017). 'Assessment of caregiving constructs: toward a personal, familial, group, and cultural construction of dementia care through the eyes of personal construct psychology.' *Journal of Cross-Cultural Gerontology 32* (4), 413–431.

Harris, P.B. and Keady, J. (2009). 'Selfhood in younger onset dementia: transitions and testimonies.' *Aging and Mental Health 13* (3), 437–444.

Healthtalk (2019). *Carers of People with Dementia: Becoming a Carer.* Accessed on 29/3/20 at https://healthtalk.org/carers-people-dementia/becoming-a-carer.

Ignatieff, M. (1993). *Scar Tissue.* New York: Farrar, Straus and Giroux.

Johannessen, A., Engedal, K. and Thorsen, K. (2015). 'Adult children with young onset dementia narrate their experiences of their youth through metaphors.' *Journal of Multidisciplinary Healthcare 8*, 245–254.

Kyngäs, H., Mikkonen, R., Nousiainen, E., Rytilahti, M., Seppänen, P., Vaattovaara, R. and Jämsa, T. (2001). 'Coping with the onset of cancer: coping strategies and resources of young people with cancer.' *European Journal of Cancer Care 10* (1), 6–11.

Lee, S., Roen, K. and Thornton, A. (2014). The psychological impact of a diagnosis of Alzheimer's disease. *Dementia 13* (3), 289–305.

Leggett, A., Polenick, C., Maust, D. and Kales, H. (2018). 'What Hath Night to Do with Sleep? The caregiving context and dementia caregivers' nighttime awakenings.' *Clinical Gerontologist 41*, 158–166.

Lishman, E., Cheston, R. and Smithson, J. (2016). 'The paradox of dementia: changes in assimilation after receiving a diagnosis.' *Dementia 15* (2), 181–203.

Luft, J. and Ingham, H. (1955). *The Johari Window: A Graphic Model for Interpersonal Relations.* University of California: Western Training Lab.

MacKinlay, E. (2012). 'Belief and ageing: spiritual pathways in later life.' *Australasian Journal on Ageing 31*, 2.

Maslow, A. (1954). *Motivation and Personality.* New York: Harper and Row Publishers.

Maslow, A. (1970). *Motivation and Personality (2nd edition).* New York: Harper and Row Publishers.

McSherry, W. and Smith, J. (2012). 'Spiritual care.' In W. McSherry, R. McSherry and R. Watson (eds) *Care in Nursing. Principles, Values and Skills.* Oxford: Oxford University Press.

Morris, G. and Morris, J. (2010). *The Dementia Care Workbook.* Buckingham: Open University Press.

Narayanasamy, A. (2010). 'Recognising spiritual needs.' In W. McSherry and L. Ross (eds) *Spiritual Assessment in Healthcare Practice.* Keswick: M&K Publishing.

National Alliance for Caregiving (NAC). Accessed on 31/1/20 at www.caregiving.org.

Nichols, K., Fam, D., Cook, C., Pearce, M., Elliot, G., Baago, S., Rockwood, K. and Chow, T. (2013). 'When dementia is in the house: needs assessment survey for young caregivers.' *Canadian Journal of Neurological Sciences 40* (1), 21–28.

Pratchett, T. (2008). '"A butt of my own jokes": Terry Pratchett on the disease that finally claimed him.' 15 March. Accessed on 15/12/10 at www.theguardian.com/books/2015/mar/15/a-butt-of-my-own-jokes-terry-pratchett-on-the-disease-that-finally-claimed-him.

Prior, B. and Drummond, M. (2018). *Grandma and Me: A Kid's Guide for Alzheimer's and Dementia.* London: Morgan James Publishing.

Robinson, L., Clare, L. and Evans, K. (2005). 'Making sense of dementia and adjusting to loss: psychological reactions to a diagnosis of dementia in couples.' *Aging and Mental Health 9*, 337–347.

Robinson L., Gemski, A., Abley, C., Bond, J., Keady, J., Campbell, S., Samsi, K. and Manthorpe, J. (2011). 'The transition to dementia – individual and family experiences of receiving a diagnosis: a review.' *International Psychogeriatrics 23* (7), 1026–1043.

Russell, P. and Johnston, N. (2017). *Grandma Forgets.* Chatswood, Australia: EK Books.

Shim, B., Barroso, J., Gilliss, C. and Davis, L. (2013). 'Finding meaning in caring for a spouse with dementia.' *Applied Nursing Research 26* (3), 121–126.

Strawbridge, W. and Wallhagen, M. (1991). 'Impact of family conflict on adult child caregivers.' *The Gerontologist 31*, 770–777.

Svanberg, E., Stott, J. and Spector, A. (2010). '"Just helping": children living with a parent with young onset dementia.' *Aging and Mental Health 14* (6), 740–751.

Swaffer, K. (2016). *What the Hell Happened to My Brain? Living Beyond Dementia.* London: Jessica Kingsley Publishers.

World Health Organization (2017). *Global Action Plan on the Public Health Response to Dementia 2017–2025.* Geneva: World Health Organization. Accessed on 16/9/18 at www.who.int/mental_health/neurology/dementia/action_plan_2017_2025/en.

Yalom, I. (2005). *The Theory and Practice of Group Psychotherapy (5th Edition).* New York: Basic Books.

Young Dementia UK (2019). *Ken H's Story.* Accessed on 15/8/19 at www.youngdementiauk.org/ken-hs-story.

Zeisl, J. (2010). *I'm Still Here. Creating a Better Life for a Loved One Living with Alzheimer's.* London: Piatkus.

Chapter 5

Struggling

Introduction

Central features within this chapter address the more difficult and distressing aspects connected with the dementia experience such as loss and despair and their detrimental impact upon personal and family dynamics. We can regard these issues as occurring across holistic dimensions affecting individuals' lives through multi-faceted ways. For the person with dementia, the steady deterioration of function can be marked with progressive restrictions as their sphere of occupation and engagement steadily shrinks. Enforced dependency can be a particularly difficult aspect to accept as personal autonomy becomes constrained, for example having to stop driving and its striking effect upon a person's self-esteem and individual sphere of freedom. Increased dependence upon others will impact upon family and friends with common reports of fatigue, stress, detachment from social and work interests and a relegation of personal needs. This can evoke mixed feelings amongst carers and family members including tension and resentment directed towards the person being cared for or others who are perceived as not 'pulling their weight'. The devastating feelings of separation and isolation, experienced by those with dementia and their family members, are clearly difficult to cope with as their social sphere gradually becomes more constricted. Perhaps the most potent and frightening of the losses experienced is that of self, causing extreme distress to all family members. It is important to note that whilst this chapter retains a focus upon the more difficult and depressing elements of the dementia experience it only features part of the overall journey, which in total represents a fluidly changing dynamic between points of both struggling and coping.

The story so far

The Lawrences have started to individually and collectively consider what the presence of dementia within their family signifies for them. It involves attempting to find acceptance and optimism for a condition that commonly carries such negative and devastating connotations. This heralds changes for all concerned including a reorganization of roles and responsibilities as well as contemplating the giving up or restricting of occupational and social pursuits. The family are in essence attempting to negotiate their way through this maze and prepare themselves for the tempestuous times ahead.

Chapter themes

This chapter will introduce the reader to the following themes:

- The burden of dementia – 'It's all becoming too much'
- Identity crisis and loss of self – 'I am disappearing'
- Isolation and separateness – 'We are feeling very alone'
- Despair – 'The future looks bleak'

The burden of dementia ('It's all becoming too much')

This section highlights the growing strain that is being felt by the whole family, with members feeling increasingly irritable, unsettled and drained, emotionally as well as physically. It also highlights the relentless *and* unceasing nature of difficulties encountered within their dementia experience. The holistic nature of this experience was documented by Diana Friel McGowin (1994) in her book *Living in the Labyrinth: A Personal Journey Through the Maze of Alzheimer's,* which described the emotional, physical and social turmoil that Alzheimer's had on her life and her family. This at times became all-encompassing, placing immense strain upon the functioning of individual members and the family as a whole. The nature of the burden experienced by those concerned is explored in the following section as relating to:

- the person with dementia
- carers and family members.

Person with dementia

Peter's Narrative 5.1: Contemplating life

'It has been a while now since I was given my diagnosis and my thoughts are becoming trapped between what life used to be for me and what it is likely to be like in the future. As for my family and social life, they continue to pose challenges and I am especially struggling to occupy my time in any meaningful activities. Just living my normal day-to-day life feels a struggle and I know I am slowly becoming more of a burden to others. I am not working and don't really see that I am contributing anything of value to the family.

I feel lonely at times and am becoming increasingly more remote and separate from Gill – and yet we share most days together. If I could just feel more in control and on top of things then maybe I could cope with my negative moods.'

- *What thoughts and feelings are you observing from Peter's narrative? You may find it helpful to consider your responses alongside the following sub-headings:*
  - *Peter's self and well-being*
  - *Peter as a father and a husband*
  - *Peter as a contributor to the family.*

Peter's narrative highlights the growing strain that his dementia experience is having upon him. It illustrates how his thoughts have become centred around the changes forced upon him as well as projected future difficulties. His ruminations are also concerned with the burden that he is steadily becoming to others. The sense and comprehension of 'burden' can relate to a number of issues including the strain felt through demands being placed upon a person's processing faculties. This can leave individuals feeling drained and despairing, helpless in the face of their increasing difficulties. As noted by Alzheimer's Disease International (2019), tiredness within dementia can be caused by the process of feeling overwhelmed by what one is attending to. Studies have shown that the increase in dementia severity is matched with a corresponding decrease in a person's cognitive functionality (Nebes and Brady 1992; Stephens *et al.* 2004). It is not surprising therefore to note that this impacted cognitive ability will pose many daily challenges for those affected.

If thinking about our own lives, we can consider how frustrating it is when struggling to make sense of what others are saying to us if maybe information is spoken too quickly or poorly articulated. We can also reflect upon how we feel when asking passers-by for directions and becoming lost in their wordy or convoluted responses. Such incidents can be passed off as irritants with alternative means sought to deal with them. If this, however, becomes an increasingly regular occurrence and our capacity to deal with such issues is compromised, we can appreciate that we would begin to struggle. Research by Hart and Wells (1997) showed heightened agitation when instructions were given to residents (with dementia) at a complexity level above their comprehension ability. Matching instruction complexity to language comprehension of those with dementia was found to reduce agitation. This illustrates the personal reaction to what can feel bewildering, demeaning and incomprehensible, or simply leaving one feeling 'stupid'. The dynamics reflect a process whereby carers may be ignorant of the internal dynamics, attributing a person's lack of response to their deteriorating cognition. The focus can be more intently applied to a person's behaviour, with a nursing home resident, 'George', for example, noted as being agitated and restless without considering what his corresponding feelings might be.

The affected processing time within the dementia experience is reflected by Wendy Mitchell (2018), in relation to her daily life. Driving, an activity she previously engaged in with a fair degree of comfort, had become very difficult and she related subsequently feeling startled, unsafe and bewildered as to why her brain was unable to make the necessary computations. Another incident that took her by surprise related to a meeting at work when she found herself suddenly at a loss for words, unable to articulate what she wished to relate. This left her feeling shameful, stupid, frustrated, confused and humiliated. Likewise, a participant in Haak's study (2002) about communication in people with dementia related: 'When I try to speak, I see what I'm going to say in my mind, and then the words turn around and go further and further out of sight… So I don't say anything.'

Such incidents convey powerfully the sense of helplessness and shock felt when a person is suddenly faced with an inability to process and respond to situations that in earlier times would have been dealt with fairly comfortably and automatically. The experienced sensory overload can also leave individuals feeling drained, physically as well as emotionally. This is seen in Robert Davis's (1989, p.99) narrative with a very expressive report about the demands upon his processing faculties through the excess stimulation encountered during a family trip to Disney World:

> The rides with their blinking and flashing lights. The confusion of the crowds, the long wait in line, totally exhausted my reserves. I needed to go to the

> room and lie down… I lay in a dark room listening to the tapes that keep my mind from falling into the 'black hole', that tries to suck me in every time I stop concentrating on something.

It took him weeks following this experience to recoup his ability to adequately function. Davis (1989) was able to comprehend and articulate the reason for his fatigue although he acknowledged that earlier on in the dementia journey exhaustion can be mistakenly attributed to other factors such as work stress or ageing. With this in mind, we can reflect upon the pressure that individuals of working age might encounter before they have a diagnosis with which to appreciate what is causing them to feel exhausted. Within a younger, working age group, this can advance the potential for misdiagnosis, particularly as early signs of dementia, including fatigue and poor concentration, can mimic those of depression (Nazarko 2009).

It is not surprising that over a prolonged period of time, struggling with cognitive processing can cause a person to withdraw from activities and social contact. The response from others including family and friends can be to assume that a person's withdrawal and relegation of activities is a sign of their dwindling abilities and erosion of independence, with 'well-meaning' carers subsequently stepping up their involvement of helping. The potentially destructive nature of this is outlined in Kitwood's (1997) description of *malignant social psychology*, for example disempowerment and invalidation and changes in relationship power dynamics. Part of the problem lies with carers and family members struggling or feeling unable to communicate with the person with dementia. If we properly attend though to what individuals with dementia are telling us we might begin to pick out their desires or instructions as to how they would like others to respond and what aids them to cope with the burden upon their deteriorating cognitive processing abilities:

- Questions and instructions should be provided at a pace that can be comfortably accessed.
- Understand and make allowances for what a person might struggle with.
- Allow time to rest and recover.
- Recognize what a person can still do.
- Look for ways to assist with difficulties (including creative modes of expression).

Wendy Mitchell (2019) reflects upon the immense organization and time to complete activities that her dementia requires to be attended to on a daily basis. It is not helped by having an 'invisible disability' and she reflects that: 'strangers don't understand if we can't get through a door quick enough because the black mass in front of us looks like a hole.'

Her exertions frequently left her with a 'banging headache', although her determination to retain her independence and not lose her abilities provided the impetus to maintain her self-coping. Kitwood (1997), building around the work of Bender and Cheston (1997), examined the dementia experience in relation to the continued demands upon a person's processing functions and the domain of negative experiences:

- *Feelings.* Associated with specific emotions such as frustration or uselessness at being unable to carry out everyday tasks. These feeling states are available to people when cognitive impairment is relatively slight.
- *Global states.* Include 'raw emotions', including terror, misery or rage unattached to specific situations. This also includes general confusion and may accompany high or low levels of arousal.
- *'Burn-out' states.* Occurs when a person's nervous system has been in a high level of arousal for a long period leaving them severely depleted.

ACTIVITY 5.1

Consider what Peter's burdens could be.

What might Peter think the family feel towards him?

A person is likely to travel across this domain on a number of occasions with functionality progressively impacted upon, although as Kitwood (1997) asserts, with the right level of support including psychotherapy, one can be assisted to cope with the changes taking place and one's emotional response to these.

Another element to consider is anticipated future burdens, especially if becoming less independent and requiring care input from family members. Fears and worries about this can be heightened by the alteration that this can bring within relationships and roles within a family. As Wendy Mitchell (2018, p.68) reflected: 'I never want you to be my carers. You're my daughters and always will be.'

Listening to these words we can only imagine the sense of desperate helplessness and fear felt as individuals contemplate their future, desiring support from people who love them and who are able to represent their needs yet conscious of the demands and pressures that they will over time place upon others. Similarly, DeBaggio (2002, p.58) articulated his worries for the future and the impact that his decreased abilities and independence was likely to have upon his family: 'I only have a few years before I become a hatstand.'

This is also powerfully expressed in terms of his awareness about the continued distress endured by his family on account of him and his deteriorating condition (DeBaggio 2002, p.121): 'Alzheimer's hit them as surely as it has hit me. They are reluctant to reveal their pain and fear to me but every time they see me or talk to me they must be reminded of their own sorrow.'

This will clearly cause the person severe distress to feel that they are, albeit inadvertently, the cause of such sadness in others.

Carers and family members

Gill's Narrative 5.2: Stress and fatigue

'There is no let-up with this bloody dementia. I just feel so completely drained and am desperate for a bit of respite. I can't think of when I get any space for myself during the day as Peter's needs are just so unpredictable. Night times are hardly any better as I am on tenterhooks listening out for any sounds that Peter has got up. He doesn't sleep very well and gets particularly distressed if he wakes in the night without anyone to reassure him. He is restless and agitated for most of the day too. He has said how useless he feels and he does get very angry with himself for what he sees as his failings.

We are ratty and irritable with each other fairly much all the time. Ashleigh seems impatient and short-tempered. Matt just does not want to know, getting irritable whenever any of our struggles are raised. Even Tom who is usually so easy going is very moody with me and quick to get angry. His school tutor has invited me in for a meeting about him as his grades are still dropping and she is worried that the stress at home is inhibiting his concentration on school work.

I don't have any time for myself now or opportunities to recharge my already depleted batteries. I feel utterly exhausted and drained emotionally and spiritually. There is not much left to give yet what can I do?'

- *Consider what Gill's dementia burdens could be.*
- *What might Gill feel the family needs to talk about?*

Gill's narrative continues to express emotional turmoil with the whole family feeling 'trapped' within Peter's dementia. The impression given is of feeling suffocated, striving to meet the demands of being a wife and mother yet starved of personal space and deprived of healthy respite throughout her day. The stress and burden of caring varies greatly according to a multitude of factors, which also relates to the type of dementia involved. As Lee *et al.* (2013) found, those caring for individuals with dementia with Lewy bodies or Parkinson's dementia experienced more stress than those caring for persons with Alzheimer's disease and vascular dementia. Carer stress was associated with higher levels of psychosis, mood disturbances, daytime sleep and cognitive fluctuations in the person with dementia. This highlights factors associated with behaviours that are taxing and disturbing of carers' well-being.

Activity 5.2 provides a 'burdens of care' matrix by highlighting three health planes, some bullet points have been left vacant for you to complete.

ACTIVITY 5.2

Physical health	**Emotional health**
• Tiredness • Poor sleep patterns • .... •	• Anger vs guilt feelings • Caring vs feelings of being 'trapped' • .... • ....
Burden(s) of care and their impact(s)	
What conclusions have you made about the burden of care and impact on being a carer?	**Social health** • A need for one's personal space • Respite time • .... • ....

As illustrated by Activity 5.2, caring for a family member with dementia can be an all-encompassing experience. This for many is a 24-hour, seven-days-a-week responsibility, although it is referred to by Mace and Rabins (2012) as a perceived *36-hour day* in relation to the relentless nature of one's caring role, engaged in with little or no respite. The soul-destroying nature of this experience is exacerbated by the unwelcome appearance of what Talbot (2011, p.127) calls 'end of tether' moments, which for her included an experience where she was informed that a day carer would no longer be able to assist in getting her mum up in the morning: 'I have been dreading this... Getting mum up is truly awful. She hates to get up and boy, does she let you know...looking after mum has become a nightmare. A never ending 24 hour nightmare.'

It can be both emotionally and physically exhausting, leaving carers with little energy or enthusiasm for attending to their own well-being. One's own fatigue is heightened through the relentless feelings of helplessness concerning the inability to find respite or being able to lessen the distress or plight of the cared-for family member. References to *compassion fatigue* have appeared in the literature since 1992, when the concept was first introduced to the healthcare community, with feelings of anger, inefficacy, apathy and depression resulting from a caregiver's inability to cope with devastating stress (Joinson 1992). Compassion fatigue is distinct from depression or burden involving observations of a cared-for family member's suffering. This results in feelings of helplessness, hopelessness and social isolation, minimizing a person's ability to be empathic. Day, Anderson and Davis (2014), in their study, concluded that healthcare providers, particularly nurses, are in a role to identify family caregivers at risk for compassion fatigue and provide emotional and practical support.

ACTIVITY 5.3

Linda is up before 7am to send business emails; she then takes the children to school and looks after Dad and the rest of the family for the rest of the day.

At 11pm she finally has 'me time', which she uses to run her business, before going to bed between 1am and 2am.

She is in poor physical health having low energy levels despite being on the go for 19 hours a day. Recently Linda was so exhausted that she stayed in bed until midday, which is unheard of for her.

Her husband does flexible hours and works from home providing occasional respite. She used to exercise a lot but has not been able to do much since she started to care for her dad and has put on five stone.

She has joined a gym but rarely has time to go. She would like to get a full-time job at Glasgow Airport where she previously worked but her caring responsibilities make this impossible. (Alzheimer's Research UK 2015)

What do you think this carer might be feeling?

In the case study, the effect that such an experience as Linda's might have over a series of years is perhaps hard to imagine. A stark illustration though is provided by the TV documentary *Malcolm and Barbara*. This was filmed over 11 years outlining Malcolm's declining condition and Barbara's spirit-sapping experience as his wife and carer. She speaks in the documentary of her loneliness and growing feelings of despair, and final scenes of Malcolm bedbound and virtually in a state of total dependence are heart-breaking to watch. Barbara appears totally drained and spent, with a sense of weary resignation regarding her continued plight. With such experiences being encountered it is understandable that caregiver depression will not be uncommon. The recent findings of a study by Zhu *et al.* (2015) highlighted that caregiver depressive symptoms were found to be the most consistent predictor of increases in healthcare costs over an averaged two-year period and this included costs from the use of over-the-counter drugs. What is not apparent though is the nature of support offered (besides medication) for a person's wider holistic needs.

ACTIVITY 5.4

Consider the range of activities and pastimes that fill your waking days. You might find it helpful to use sub-headings such as 'at rest', 'during play' and 'when working'.

If you are/became a carer, which of these activities would have to change or stop?

The burden of care can be widened when multiple persons are in need of support. For a significant number of carers who have a partner with young-onset dementia there can be children's needs to also attend to. Helen Beaumont (2009), caring for her husband who was diagnosed with dementia in his forties, wrote about being unable to stop and rest, having multiple responsibilities to attend to and very little time to spare. Despite breaking her Achilles tendon and having her leg plastered from toe to hip she recalls still having to attend to her husband Clive's needs whilst simultaneously looking after two primary school age children. She was heavily reliant upon friends and neighbours and negotiated with her husband's mother for respite time. This example shows how a carer's difficulties with coping can suddenly escalate but also how vital it can be having support networks within one's social circle, something many carers, especially those in older age categories do not have. There can also be a difference in the levels and type of support received from family or friends. Donnellan, Bennett and Soulsby (2017) conducted qualitative interviews with spousal dementia carers, finding the availability of friend networks more associated with resilience than support from family members, which was less matched to needs.

The caring dynamic, as well as incorporating children and other dependants, can include more than one party with dementia. Chris Carling's (2012) account *But Then Something Happened* narrates her experience of caring for both parents who had dementia. She reports a seemingly endless series of crisis events, including one she pointedly calls 'Incontinence Saturday', which doesn't need much imagination to contemplate what she might have encountered and how distressing for her it would have been. Her narrative shows the relentless nature of the emotional, physical, psychological and spiritual demands that family carers have to contend with as they navigate their way through a bewildering selection of agencies and bureaucratic systems. Another person contending with both parents who had dementia, Fiona Phillips, spoke about the burden of uncertainty concerning her own future and fears about herself later developing dementia and 'disappearing' (Merriman 2015). The word 'disappearing' powerfully expresses the terrifying prospect of losing oneself within this condition with all its ravages and devastation laid bare before her eyes. We can also consider the concept of *disappearing* in terms of a family's sphere of engagement, as expressed by Carol Adams who commented about the impact that her husband's Alzheimer's has had upon their diminishing social sphere:

> Our little world is shrinking… You don't notice it at first; it happens around you. We do so much less than we used to. You have to accept that you don't want to go on that holiday or to that wedding – and you have to believe it, because otherwise you'd get upset. (*The Telegraph* 2013)

This progressive change can affect all spheres of a family's life with individuals feeling more constricted and isolated within what is felt as a 'shrinking world' (Duggan, Blackman and Martyr 2008). It can also be regarded with resignation as the above narrative shows with the expectation that this is what life now consists of.

The caring role involving multiple parties with dementia is not uncommon and as well as both parents can include other permutations including a partner and parent but, maybe also more frightening to contemplate, partner and adult child. For many people, dementia is prone to being regarded as an old person's disease and it can feel incomprehensible to acknowledge the presence of such a condition in a younger person. It seems therefore inconceivable that a parent will be confronted with one of their own children developing dementia. Kate Swaffer (n.d.) writes about her parents' burden of sadness concerning her dementia diagnosis with her mother relating:

> I was horrified and angry when my daughter told me she had dementia. It was an anger that I had never felt before... There was nothing I could do. I felt so helpless. Then the anger subsided and I was left with a feeling of deep, deep sadness. I try to enjoy shared times together, remembering our bright energetic little girl. I cannot contemplate what lies ahead for her.

Nurse Practitioner Rita Jablonski writes a blog entitled 'Make Dementia your B*tch!' and reports upon the growing number of parents caring for adult children with dementia being seen in her clinic (MDYB 2018). Given the increasing number of people diagnosed with young-onset dementia and the progressively ageing population this is hardly surprising. Kate Swaffer's narrative above illustrates what an unexpected shock this can be with deep feelings of rage and injustice.

The burden of care can be widened to encompass the whole holistic domain, which also includes a person's financial struggle. It is alarming to note the Carers UK (2010) report that a significant number of carers are missing out on millions of pounds of unclaimed Carer's Allowance. Inspirational campaigner, Annie Dransfield, a former Carers UK trustee and 2013 *Yorkshire Evening Post* Carer of the Year, has an extensive caring role, at one point involving full-time care for her disabled son as well as an elderly parent with dementia. She reflected: 'I am caring over 35 hours a week. You are on call 24-7, it's a full-time job and more. I stopped teaching several years ago to care full time because my son's needs became more complex.'

She was very critical of government policy around benefit entitlements, which resulted in many carers not claiming their weekly entitlements because of the cared-for person having their own allowances deducted (*Yorkshire Evening Post* 2013). This illustrates a very real problem with the benefits system and fails to properly acknowledge the dilemma felt by well-meaning carers who are influenced to again relegate their own needs. The fact that carers are saving the UK health and social services over £57 billion yearly (Alzheimer's Society 2017) through their input should be properly recognized. In the authors' opinion, the already overloaded health and social services would collapse without the goodwill and dedication of the hundreds of thousands involved in an unpaid caring role. It is essential therefore that there be a proper investment in terms of support for this multitude of carers.

When trying to encapsulate what a *caring burden* might entail, there are a number of terms we might encounter including 'stress', 'despair' and 'helplessness'. These words do not do justice though to what a person's lived experience, including all the corresponding thoughts and emotions, might entail. Andrea Gillies (2009) cared for her mother-in-law with Alzheimer's and wrote about 'stress' as a protectively imprecise term, preferring that of 'incompatibility'. This had a debilitating physical impact upon her, experiencing 'funny turns' with the sensation of the room spinning, her head swirling and feeling nauseous, all of which eventually prevented her from any further activity and confined her to periods in bed. It appears here as if the person's body is taking charge and incapacitating them through a homeostatic attempt to protect the individual and restore function.

ACTIVITY 5.5

What does the phrase 'respite care' mean for you?

Is your definition based upon personal or professional experience?

What are the merits or not of providing respite care for the person?

Respite

Marianne Talbot (2011) took her mother with dementia into her own home to help care for her. Her periods of respite when her brothers shared some of the caring illustrated the ongoing repression of her own needs. She describes then feeling a 'free agent' spending her time playing music at full volume, tending her garden (without having to simultaneously find ways to keep her mum occupied), having friends to visit, going out for meals or watching films without interruptions or added commentary. This narrative expressed very strongly the craving for personal space, something which allows us time to attend to our own well-being needs, which is essential in terms of our ongoing ability to cope. However, finding respite can also be met with further stresses as Talbot (2011) recounted, after her mum spent a week in a care home. Her mother returned at the end of the week traumatized, filthy and missing clothing items as well as her teeth. Her week's respite was followed by five arduous weeks of consoling and soothing her mum. She also writes about her burden of despair concerning the thought of her mum being in a home full-time, lost and alone, which subsequently led her to cancel all future respite care. Similarly, Barbara despaired at the genuinely distressed state her husband Malcolm returned in following his short respite care, feeling that it wholly undermined the time she had for herself, causing more problems (*Malcolm and Barbara* 2007).

Young family members

Young people respond to such situations in different ways. They may grieve for the person with dementia as they used to be, suppress their own needs for fear of burdening other family members, or even engage in self-destructive behaviours. Whilst there can be positive aspects to young people in caring for others, research shows that young carers often experience worse outcomes than their peers in terms of health, well-being, education and income (Pakenham *et al.* 2006; Sikes 2017). Given the strain faced by young people caring for adults with dementia, statutory bodies and organizations should use and create opportunities to raise awareness about this group. Tailored information should be provided to children and young people providing care and support, and existing services should become more sensitive to the needs of families in which young people are supporting adults with dementia. Young people also need support to connect with others who share some of their experiences. The hidden numbers of young people caring for adults with dementia deserve to get the support they need so their own lives and relationships aren't undermined by the responsibilities they shoulder.

EXERCISE: CRISIS AND THE YOUNG CARER

This exercise asks you to explore personal thoughts, feelings and possible behaviours of being a 'young carer' whilst contemplating a 'life crisis'. (See Chapter 8.)

Sikes and Hall (2017) led a study exploring the perceptions and experiences of children and young people with a parent with dementia. The researchers used social media to recruit 22 young people and asked them to share their experiences of having a parent with dementia. Their findings highlighted the fact that available information and services do not offer the support needed by younger family members. They also illustrated that the education and careers of young people can be negatively affected, with them experiencing difficulties around concentrating, work and school hours, and in pursuing higher education. Their personal lives were also affected by their parents' dementia, with parents missing their significant life events, such as graduations and weddings. They also felt they could no longer rely on their parents for help or advice, or have them involved in their life decisions. Some also experienced jealousy of their friends who had parents with conditions that are no longer stigmatized and for which treatment may be available, such as cancer.

A survey by the National Children's Bureau (2016) found many young people reluctant to take on the role and identity of a 'carer', feeling that they were not doing enough to help, which reveals a feeling recognized by Svanberg, Stott and Spector (2010) as being unable to fulfil the role expected of them. Research undertaken for the Department for Education concluded that young carers known to local services did identify with the term 'young carer'. Young carers were proud of their caring role but also recognized that it was used as a label that carried with it negative connotations. Young carers not receiving formal support services did not self-identify with the term 'young carer' and parents of these children and young people expressed concerns about their child being labelled as a young carer, a label which they felt reflected negatively on them as a parent.

The findings above highlight very clearly some of the difficulties and stressors encountered by young carers with very distinct support needs reflected.

Identity crisis and loss of self ('I am disappearing')

This section concerns what is perhaps the most frightening element to contemplate when diagnosed with dementia, that of losing *self*. We can regard the concept of self and possession of personal narratives as immensely powerful signifiers of existence. Descartes' (Open University 2015) Latin proposition *cogito ergo sum* (I think, therefore I am) shows the contemplation of one's existence proving that an 'I' exists to do the thinking. As cognitive abilities dwindle, so too do fears increase that self may become lost. The devastatingly crushing fear shared by many people of losing self is captured by Fiona Phillips' fears in the previous section, about simply *disappearing*. This captures the personal devastation commonly felt in relation to the sense of vanishing and simply ceasing to exist. It is a fear that extends to other family members with the devastation of 'losing' the person within their condition of dementia. Dupuis' (2002) study examined the experience of ambiguous loss for family members caring for a person with dementia. This involved several phases including *anticipatory loss, progressive loss* and *acknowledged loss*. Acceptance and avoidance were the two most common coping strategies used in dealing with acknowledged loss. This will all be examined in depth within this section.

Gill's Narrative 5.3: I am losing Peter

'I feel like I am losing Peter or the essence of who he is and it is utterly heart-breaking. The fact that Peter has periods where he is very cognisant of this just tears me apart. Watching Peter sobbing and despairing about what he terms as "slipping away" is just too painful to bear. The only consolation about his dementia is that he does sometimes lose his awareness about all of this. I don't though!

There seems to be a fair bit of acknowledgement about the loss of identity for those affected with dementia. What about our identity as a couple, or as a whole family? Who really acknowledges that apart from those directly affected? Our family unity is being torn apart and crushed through this blasted illness. My husband and children's father is fading from our midst and there is nothing we can do to prevent it.'

- *What are your thoughts about Gill's narrative?*
- *If you could offer advice/support to Gill and the family at the present time, what would it be?*

Gill's narrative outlines her feeling of despair about losing Peter, or what is his essence. She uses terms such as 'slipping away' and 'loss of identity' to acknowledge what is occurring. Interestingly her concept of identity is widened to that of couple and family alongside that of Peter as an individual. There is much debate in the literature as to the extent to which self and identity persist in people with dementia. The aim of a systematic review by Cadell and Clare (2010) was to examine the persistence of self and identity throughout the course of the disease. Thirty-three studies were reviewed, which showed that many approaches have been taken to studying aspects of self and identity in dementia, including both quantitative and qualitative methods. Almost all of the studies suggest that there is at least some evidence for persistence of self in both the mild and moderate to severe stages of the illness, although many studies record some degree of deterioration in aspects of self or identity.

For the person with dementia, losing self will be a truly terrifying prospect. Christine Bryden (2018, p.21), diagnosed in her late forties, recalled the dread of: 'Hanging over me were the ominous black clouds of the loss of self that was supposed to occur with dementia.'

This journey into the unknown, heralding a gloomy and uncertain future, was eloquently summed up by the writer Iris Murdoch as 'sailing into darkness' (Nehemas 1999). We would imagine that Murdoch's gradual cognitive decline would have been truly depressing, diminishing something core to her being, namely her potent and much-celebrated ability to express herself through narrative prose. The despair that a person might feel in the contemplation of losing self is especially concerning given the enhanced risk of depression and suicide (Purandare *et al.* 2009), which is examined further later in this chapter in the section entitled 'Despair'.

The onset of memory difficulties and a diagnosis of dementia can pose a threat to how individuals view themselves with their identity struggle strongly linked to the responses of others, which may either minimize or strengthen their sense of self. Individuals can experience tensions between holding on to their identity whilst adjusting to dementia-related changes, outlined by Pearce, Clare and Pistrang (2002) as a circular process of managing an old sense of self and constructing a new one. Indeed, the literature illustrates a process of role transition with a new identity emerging through the dementia journey (Holt and Morris 2015). These changes will clearly cause difficulties for families desperate to hold on to and maintain the person they 'know'. Research by Sikes and Hall (2016) used biographical interviews to explore the experiences of 19 eight to 31-year-olds who had a parent with dementia. Their narrative accounts suggest that the construction of their parent as the same person is not helpful and that expecting them to behave and feel towards that parent as they did before is a continued source of distress. The essence of this study points to the need to support young people to the fact that their parent may well be drastically different from the mum or dad they previously knew.

This new identity though can in some instances be characterized by a lessening of inhibitions or what Kitwood (1997) identified as a loosening of psychological defences. This has the potential for individuals to feel freer and more expressive as shown in the following narrative:

> We have noticed one very positive and helpful change in my father's personality since his diagnosis. Previously he was a very shy and reserved man who found it extremely difficult to mix with other people so had little social interaction outside the family. Now this social inhibition has gone and he willingly meets new people and enjoys various clubs. This has made his care so much easier and we believe the extra stimulation has slowed down the rate of his decline. (Alzheimer's Society 2009)

This is heartening on one level although may pose problems where 'changes' are not sufficiently acknowledged or supported by carers, families and friends. As a person's communicative capacity deteriorates, their needs and wishes can be represented by what others believe they want based upon past experience. In the example above, we can imagine the added frustration, annoyance or helplessness felt if not supported with one's emergent desires and interests.

A person's awareness of their changing identity can also be regarded in the glimpses they catch of themselves from an external vantage point. Wendy Mitchell (2018, p.211) wrote about her need to remove mirrors around her house, not wanting to observe the changes taking place in her. Also, after seeing herself in a video clip on an interview, she commented: 'I didn't speak the way I used to speak, I didn't look how I remembered, and I know that as I age it will only get worse.'

Of course we might all feel startled at hearing our recorded voice or videoed image and observing ourselves from an external vantage point. However, in most cases our surprise is mild enough for us to reconcile ourselves with what we are faced with. For those with dementia the perceived changes noted can be truly shocking including instances where a person's reflection is that of an old and different person, greatly at odds with how that person feels their true self to be. Clare (2003) observed a spectrum of responses to memory deficits, ranging from self-maintaining expressions to self-adjusting ones. Faced with these tensions the individual may actively face their dementia through dealing with changes by focusing upon maintaining either their old identity or their new identity. Participants in Clare's (2003) study expressed the impact dementia had on their fundamental core and personality, occasioning attempts to maintain continuity or *holding on to self* through attending to preserved skills and compensating for losses. The process of *redefining self* involved participants moving towards identifying with their diagnosis and seeking a more robust sense of self in light of future decline.

A study by Batra, Sullivan and Geldmacher (2013) found people who were significantly impaired through dementia continuing to refer to themselves as 'I' and presenting other components indicative of self-identity. They concluded that their presentation of a coherent and continuous sense of self in discourse was very similar to non-demented age peers. Implications here concern societal views and responses to those with dementia reflecting Sabat and Harré's (1992, p.443) view that 'the primary cause of the loss of self is the ways in which others view and treat the Alzheimer's sufferer'.

This includes healthcare professionals, as reflected by studies across a range of practice settings. Dewing and Dijk (2014) highlighted that poor outcomes for people with dementia in acute hospitals result from a tension between prioritizing medical treatment and the delivery of person-centred dementia care, exacerbated by the fact that there is insufficient understanding of what person-centred care is and a lack of staff knowledge and skills to deliver such care. Clark-McGhee and Castro (2015) conducted a narrative analysis of poems from the words of people given a diagnosis of dementia. Some narratives evidenced speakers' lack of agency over their experiences, not because of the 'dementia' but due to treatment and care contexts. Other narratives demonstrated that, through acknowledging and supporting *personhood*, speakers retained a sense of well-being and purpose in their social worlds.

Sutton's (2003) paper contrasts the loss of mind from the loss of brain cells in Alzheimer's disease and other neurodegenerative conditions with the threats to one's mind from the mindlessness of others from a cognitive-analytic perspective. Case studies are presented that show how the therapeutic framework of Cognitive-Analytic Therapy (CAT), as developed by the consultant psychotherapist Anthony Ryle, can bring containment for clients facing this dilemma, particularly when past trauma is potentially overwhelming (Ryle 1997). This is set in a dialogue with Kitwood's concept of *malignant social psychology* being restated in terms of *reciprocal roles* as developed in CAT.

Bryden (2018, p.34) illustrates her deteriorating sense of time, recall and language yet still being able to acknowledge a sense of self and: 'I can still reflect on meaning… I can explore my experience in the present moment and reflect upon my unfolding narrative to discover a continuing sense of self, within my changing experiences of and interactions with the world.'

Figure 5.1 provides an approach for reflecting on past and present factors as ways of developing/maintaining/losing 'self and identity'. The two prompts of 'who' and 'what' in both segments ask you to consider relationships between your self, other people and the environment(s) you live in.

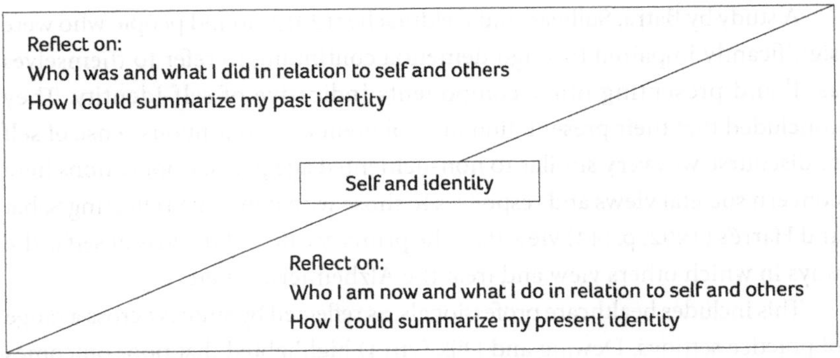

Figure 5.1 Identity and stigma

Reframing of identity and stigma

Goffman (1963, p.3) defines stigma as a sign or mark that designates the possessor as 'spoiled' and therefore as less valued than 'normal' people; it is: 'deeply discrediting' and reduces the bearer 'from a whole and usual person to a tainted, discounted one'. An extension of Goffman's description by Benbow and Jolley (2012) suggests that stigma involves the three aspects of discrimination, stereotypes and prejudice.

ACTIVITY 5.6

Figure 5.1 asked you to reflect on past and present factors and the ways of developing/maintaining/losing 'self and identity'.

Briefly outline how you would describe your past self (for example, when an adolescent).

Briefly describe your present self and the life events you feel have shaped your identity.

Behuniak (2011) describes the stigma labels people diagnosed with dementia may be perceived as having. These negative stereotypes highlight a loss of self and capabilities through the use of metaphors such as 'the walking dead' and 'zombies'. Link and Phelan (2001) suggest that through the process of labelling, stereotyping, separation, status loss and discrimination, stigma results in creating an 'us and them' mentality that results in 'othering' and the exclusion of one group of people by another more powerful group. A recent review on literature published between 2004 to 2015 on dementia-related stigma by Herrmann *et al.* (2018) reported that the severity of stigmatizing attitudes is shaped by a number of factors that include age, gender, personal experience, profession, ethnicity, culture, beliefs, understandings of prognosis and experience with persons living with dementia. The review also noted that there was no published accepted 'gold standard' for assessing or reducing stigma, either in dementia literature or the broader stigma literature.

Milne (2010, p.228) considered relationships between stigma, discrimination and dementia, asserting that persons with dementia may become vulnerable to assuming a stigmatized identity as dementia 'confers a "master status" on the individual "having dementia", not only becomes the most prominent aspect of the person's life but it also serves to subsume all their other attributes and features'.

Furthermore, Mitchell, Dupuis and Kontos (2013, p.4) wrote:

> Once diagnosed with dementia, persons and their feelings, actions, and expressions become symptoms within a problematized field of possibility. If persons with dementia express feeling healthy and well, they are judged as being in denial. If they are having trouble remembering details but fill in the gaps to save face, they are said to be confabulating. If they get angry with the way in which healthcare workers are providing care, then they are labelled as aggressive and may end up being restrained and isolated.

This is a fairly damning statement showing how the person is reduced to their psychopathology and exhibited behaviours. Sabat and Harré (1992), in describing the social construction of dementia, argued that a sense of self is still retained by the person but the public sense of self can be lost if others fail to acknowledge it. Their work concluded that the attitudes and behaviours shown by other people can negate the person's sense of self if they ignore or demean it. In more recent times and specifically within South Asian families, Mackenzie (2006) argued that the stigma of dementia within family carer groups was tending to be linked to religious beliefs. A consequence was that dementia could bring about fear and jeopardize family honour and reputation, where symptoms were seen as evidence of a powerful curse.

In terms of descriptive imagery relating to the person with dementia, Shenk (2003) provides the metaphor of the slow and steady 'reverse childhood', a powerfully evocative statement. He also offers the following:

> Imagine your backwards teenager traversing her way back to infancy, to her

> very first day of birth, her first breath, and you have a surprisingly good grasp of the unravelling mind, soul, and body that Alzheimer's inflicts on the person. Every skill, feeling, and fact that the patient has learned slowly, satisfyingly, is being steadily erased as if by some sort of cosmic punishment. (Shenk 2003, p.126)

Whilst this conceptualization of reverse childhood or 'unlearning' can explain something of what is being experienced, it is important to also retain focus upon the essential person that still exists. For example, in direct contrast to a man with dementia's son who regarded his father as a shadow of the man he used to be, Rabbi Cary Kozberg (n.d.) referred to this same individual as:

> One of the most spiritually alive people I know... Dementia may steal the mind but it cannot encroach upon the soul. In my work I see how alive and vibrant the soul can remain, even when a person's cognitive capacities are significantly diminished.

Such a view upon retained personhood helps to combat infantilizing care approaches, which can emerge through processes such as Kitwood's (1997) *malignant social psychology*.

Isolation and separateness ('We are feeling very alone')

Isolation is a depressingly common experience for those with dementia, carers and family members as their worldly spheres progressively shrink. Feelings of loneliness and disconnection are experienced in relation to losses across a number of contexts such as work, social activities, friendships and family. Hawkley and Cacioppo (2010, p.218) have defined loneliness as: 'a distressing feeling that accompanies the perception that one's social needs are not being met by the quantity or especially the quality of one's social relationships'.

Loss of social roles can occur through people being unable to live up to previously held roles, or having roles taken away (Ettema *et al.* 2007). This steady experience of disengagement can be down to the person with dementia and family members withdrawing themselves or the struggle others might find in knowing how to relate and communicate with them. In society, our request to others about their well-being is usually transmitted with the expectation of them responding that they are 'fine' or else only temporarily incapacitated, to which we can offer our best wishes for a 'speedy recovery'. It is much more challenging and taxing when a person's health problems are enduring or continuing to deteriorate. In such instances offering meaningful support can be difficult to do, especially if holding the attitude that those affected are 'not going to get better'. A further issue to consider concerns the difficulties in communicating with those who are losing their ability to express themselves with coherent and understandable words. Such issues can leave well-wishers feeling dispirited and helpless, having the effect of reducing one's contact, which can become less frequent and for shorter periods. To some extent this can be regarded as a self-protective response with individuals seeking to minimize their own feelings of awkwardness and impotence at being unable to help. The following section explores these issues in more detail including the detrimental and restrictive resonance that they have upon those with dementia and their families' daily experiences.

Gill's Narrative 5.4: Feeling lonely

'I am starting to feel very alone and lost. Most days go by without seeing anyone who is not connected with the health services. Our friends seem to have stopped visiting or else have to leave after only the briefest of stays. I can hardly blame them, I suppose, as I can see they feel uneasy and unsure of what to say. It does feel a relief though when they leave as for most of their visit I am simply willing Peter to be on one of his better days. Consequently I am not able to relax.

Practically, friends have been very helpful, offering to do shopping and other such things. What I long for though is someone to sit and really connect with me and Peter in a meaningful way. I just feel as if we are becoming invisible and fading away.'

■ *If you were one of these friends, in what ways could you 'really connect'?*

Gill's narrative evokes the sense of detachment and disengagement felt from close acquaintances with others gradually disappearing from their lives. Cahill, O'Shea and Pierce (2012) in a research review for Ireland's national dementia strategy commented that the carers of people with dementia believe that society does not want to engage with or hear about people with dementia, and this leads to feelings of desperation and a lack of support for both the person with dementia and their family. As articulated by Kate Swaffer (2016, p.152):

> I am not so sure the loneliness of dementia is any worse than when you are facing any other terminal disease or major crisis, except that the stigma and

> discrimination of dementia exacerbates the loneliness as so many cannot seem to get over their own fear of the disease and subsequently stop visiting us.

This, according to Swaffer, can leave families feeling 'gagged', unable to share more distressing feelings and fears about their mortality with the sense that others don't want to or can't bear to consider them. This is a hugely significant statement and illustrates a core difficulty encountered by many families, feeling discouraged by others who are desirous of maintaining more upbeat and less uncomfortable conversations. The experience of *isolation* can be regarded as a broadly encompassing term, something Robert Davis (1989, p.97) recounted as more than simply being out of contact with others, instead concerned with feelings of disconnectedness and detachment:

> There are times when I feel normal. At other times I cannot follow what is going on around me, as the conversation whips too fast from person to person and before I have processed one comment, the thread has moved to another person or another topic, and I am left isolated from the action – alone in a crowd.

This sense of being 'alone in a crowd' is a powerfully evocative experience as articulated by Swaffer (2013a; 2013b) and DeBaggio (2002, p.200): 'Even when I am with people laughing with them, I am alone, isolated from the normal world… I live in a strange place of isolation.'

Such narratives are expressive of a spiritual detachment evoking a sense of a person existing in a bubble or vacuum separated from others by a barrier. The separation from other people can be internally generated as well as being instigated through external factors. A participant in Haak's (2002) study reflects how a person can disengage through a lessening of their confidence when in social arenas. This addresses an important point and reminds us that merely including those with dementia in group activities does not necessarily address the problem of isolation, which could be regarded as more about disengagement and disconnectedness. This was reflected by participants in Duane, Brasher and Koch's (2011) study, who saw loneliness as distinct from experiences of living alone. Indeed, Weiss (1973) proposed two theoretically distinct forms of loneliness:

- *social isolation* – absence of engaging social networks (friends, family and acquaintances)
- *emotional isolation* – absence of a close emotional attachment (e.g. partner).

The loss of emotional attachment is commonly experienced alongside social isolation by carers as reflected by Dixey (2016) in relation to her partner Irene's dementia causing the loss of her 'soul mate'. She treasured moments, when visiting her partner in a care facility when they could cuddle up together and feel connected. Her account highlights the potency of separateness felt through loss of intimacy, which can be regarded as spiritually eroding. Whilst her expressions of affection and closeness were supported by care home staff there are many accounts of gay carers feeling disregarded and side-lined. Harrison (2001) comments upon the 'heteronormativity' of care services, which compounds the feelings of invisibility of older lesbians and gay men. Clearly, intimacy and closeness are central to individuals' well-being but are often clumsily related to within healthcare settings, responded to with uncertainty or high levels of guardedness and embarrassment. In Archibald's (2003) study, staff discomfiture with sexuality was marked by concerns around residents' capacity or competence for consent, but also applied ageism and the construction of older people as asexual. Whilst capacity and consent are highly important factors, we should also be cognisant of the potential to further deny individuals opportunities for expression of what lies at the core of their being. Ward *et al.*'s (2005) study noted differences in how sexual expression is regarded within care homes according to gender, with men more often deemed by care workers to be problematic and women prone to unwelcome advances. Masculine transgression commonly evoked a punishing response, including discharge from a home or removal to other areas of a care facility.

In terms of intimacy, a powerful means of connectedness is through the sense of *touch*. A hugely illustrative example is provided by Naomi Feil, developer of the validation approach. This involved her interaction with Gladys Wilson, a lady with dementia who appeared to have retreated inwardly and to be beyond any meaningful connection. Feil's approach was very engaging, holding Gladys' hand, stroking her cheeks and arms and tapping in rhythm with her. The breakthrough came:

> At one point where she got very quiet and peaceful, and my voice became very quiet and peaceful as hers and my breathing slowed to her breathing, she pulled me to her and I moved with her and for her at that moment I believe I was a symbol of her mum. (Memory Bridge 2009, YouTube, 3.44)

This approach evoked memories and experiences connected with attachment as relating to Bowlby's (1997) conceptual model. For Gladys, the potent sense of reconnection with this maternal symbol will clearly be soothing and nurturing and help to decrease her sense of separateness and isolation.

In Moyle, Kellett and Ballantyne's (2011, p.1449) research, some carers associated memory loss with an enhanced susceptibility to loneliness. Other carers, however, considered the symptoms of memory loss as ameliorating feelings of loneliness:

> They don't comprehend. It does take away a lot of the problems with loneliness. Her short-term memory loss would help a little bit. If I said to her 'do you feel lonely at the moment?'...then a couple of minutes later she wouldn't.

Central to this theme is the perception that cognitive dysfunction is similarly connected with emotional experience, as if feeling is dependent upon thinking. This fails to acknowledge the opportunities for people with advancing dementia to feel joy as well as despair. Haak (2002) relates a dynamic of communicative isolation experienced along with the assumption that persons with dementia's communication is devoid of meaning and that they are unable to comprehend what others are expressing. Such attitudes serve to strengthen the barrier between those with dementia and others. Once such an assumption has been made, attention can be placed more strongly upon a person's externalized behaviour as opposed to reaching out and trying to connect with their internal lived experience. Reducing our attempts to connect at a meaningful level with those with dementia is liable to result in them retreating further inwards, away from a world that is becoming increasingly more incomprehensible and unfathomable. Such a retreat and reinforced disconnectedness will place the person in a desperately lonely place. Being cognisant of this does not in itself help, as many carers and family members will, through fatigue and variable levels of understanding, struggle to properly 'attend' to the person with dementia.

Isolation amongst dementia carers is very common and according to Carers UK (2015), 83 per cent of carers have felt lonely or socially isolated as a result of their caring responsibilities. The experience of disengagement can be a progressive experience as highlighted by Alzheimer's Research UK (2015) and the example of Donald who cares for his wife Lillian. They rarely go out and are isolated from friends and family with him discouraging them from visiting, regarding Lillian as his responsibility. This they reflect on as common to many male carers who feel reluctant to describe themselves as carers or seek support with their caring role. Brodaty and Hadzi-Pavlovic (2009) surveyed members of the Alzheimer's Disease and Related Disorders Society, confirming high rates of social isolation in family carers of persons with dementia. Caregivers tended to sacrifice their leisure pursuits and hobbies, restrict time with friends and family, and to give up or reduce employment. This is shown in Michael Fassio's (2009) account of his dwindling social life and the sense of being 'grounded' as it became harder to leave his mother who had dementia. Campbell *et al.* (2008) found the strongest predictor of caregiver burden involved 'role captivity', a feeling of being trapped in one's caring role. This is compounded for lone carers where support from others and times of respite are limited. Social engagement is a vital component for well-being as shown by Lowery *et al.*'s (2000) findings that caregivers who are more satisfied with their social interactions show fewer negative psychological symptoms.

ACTIVITY 5.7

Consider the ways communication approaches can lessen a person's feelings of isolation and loneliness. You may wish to place your responses in the following sub-groups.

- visually (my body language and how I would present myself)
- verbally (the words I would use and check for understanding)
- vocally (my intonation and the ways I speak).

Minority groups

Parveen, Peltier and Oyebode (2017), in a scoping exercise on perceptions of dementia in minority ethnic communities, observed that people from BAME communities remain under-represented in specialist dementia services and are more likely to draw on those services with which they are more familiar such as religious institutions. A 2011 report highlighted the need for improving support for BAME carers. One of the findings stressed that although Bangladeshis are three times more likely to be carers than white British, Bangladeshi family carers are the most deprived and neglected, and are effectively a hidden group in the UK. Geographically Bangladeshi immigrants are mostly concentrated in inner London in boroughs such as Tower Hamlets, Newham, Camden and Southwark. There are also large numbers of Bangladeshi immigrants living in Birmingham, Manchester, Oldham, Luton, Bradford, Cardiff and Portsmouth (Carers UK 2011). The isolation experienced by BME people in services in which there is little ethnic diversity and high rates of refusal to use services is among the reasons for the development of specialist culturally specific housing and care homes for BME older people with and without dementia (Moriarty, Sharif and Robinson 2011).

The problems facing minority groups can be compounded where social support is restricted as felt by a number of gay carers in terms of available family members or children. Gay carers and their partners can also feel inhibited in reaching out to mainstream services: 'We are still coming out even in our 60s. Don't want to have to keep doing that' (Rainbow Café 2018). A qualitative study by Price (2010) examined the experience carers had in 'coming out' to healthcare services. This involved a testing process of mediating disclosure of their sexuality with received responses proving a critical issue.

Despair ('The future looks bleak')

This section is concerned with the emotional toll that the experience of dementia can have upon those concerned. It involves feelings of despair and hopelessness as the contemplation of losses and future devastation upon functioning weigh heavily upon family members. This can include feelings of depression and experiences of grieving. Feelings of helplessness can be related to a variety of factors including what is being experienced, the levels of support available and opportunities to express and share one's feelings with others. The despair experienced can be far reaching and impact upon the whole family – the person with dementia, their partner and children. Hutchinson *et al.* (2016) presented data on 12 participants (aged between 19 and 33) about their experiences with a parent who has young-onset dementia. They frame the participants' emotional distress as a result of the social construction of disability, which marginalized and excluded them and their families. This can be compounded by other issues as outlined by Kate Swaffer (2016) recounting a workshop she attended relating the very varied experiences of children with parents with dementia. Some of the stories shared were of drug and alcohol abuse, homelessness and mental illness with total disengagement from the world they had known to one of invisibility and fear.

Gill's Narrative 5.5: Feeling despair

'If it wasn't for the kids I don't know if I would want to go on. Day after day of this endless torment is just too much to bear. There isn't anything to look forward to in the future except more distress and difficulty. It feels as if I am wading through treacle and seem barely alive anyway. I am completely spent and am not sure how I get through each day. There isn't even the night to gain

relief as that is nearly always disturbed and fraught with worry. I long for sleep, which I barely get, but then long for the moment when I can finally get up and gain release from the torment that my nights have become.

The family are not doing well at all with each of the children struggling. What seems unspoken between us is a secret longing to be released from this struggle – which presumably would be Peter's death. I know this makes me terribly guilty and upset and I berate myself strongly for having such thoughts.'

- *Gill's despairing thoughts and behaviours are evident. What practical suggestions could you offer? You may wish to place your responses in the following sub-groups:*
  - *personal social time and space*
  - *time and space for the children*
  - *spiritual or non-spiritual space or an equivalent faith setting*
  - *time and space with healthcare professionals.*

Gill's narrative conveys all too clearly the depth of hopelessness that can envelop a family immersed in a relentless round of difficulties day and night. A core worry given the depth of despair especially in the early days following a diagnosis is with individuals at risk of contemplating suicide (Draper *et al.* 2010). It is particularly concerning amongst a younger age group with those under 65 accounting for over a fifth of the recorded suicide cases amongst those with dementia (Purandare *et al.* 2009). From the perspective of those affected, seeking to end one's life can be regarded as an attempt to avoid the expected 'carnage' and devastation upon their lives as well as to protect family members from the burden that it is perceived they will come to place upon them. This was voiced by DeBaggio (2002, p.181):

> The day after I was diagnosed with Alzheimer's my first thought when I awoke was of suicide. I was facing a difficult, slow decline, leading to eventual loss of nearly everything human beings value, ending finally as a near-vegetable rotting in the sun.

This narrative all too painfully acknowledges the terrifying prospect of one's unremitting decline progressing towards a state of vegetation. It is unsurprising therefore to note the sense of hopelessness that can accompany such a predicted outcome. Annie Zwijnenberg, a Dutch woman with dementia, opted for euthanasia and featured in a documentary film *Before It's Too Late* (Bomford and Doyle 2019). This programme followed her progress from consultations with medical professionals through to her assisted death.

It raised, however, some debatable points about a person's capacity to make such a decision. This can be reflected against the ways in which a person's thoughts can be influenced by their mood state. The lifting, for example, of depressive symptoms and input from others can significantly alter a person's whole perspective. We can also consider the position faced whereby those who have opted for assisted death and been adjudged to have capacity may not have capacity at a later stage to confirm that this is still in line with their current wishes. Robert Davis (1989, p.23) describes the early process of his dementia transition as slowly turning his mind into a sieve that 'could only catch and hold certain random things'. In such an instance we can consider the elements that might be lost and that any decisions arrived at could be lacking in broader contemplation. His continued narrative, though, reflected: 'Even if I had every bit of my mental capacity, I still could not have dealt with this inescapable darkness.' This *inescapable darkness* reflects a sense of impotence and inability to change one's impending decline.

There are many instances where a person can be brought into contact with markers of their deteriorating faculties. Consider how you might feel in the situations posed in Activity 5.8.

ACTIVITY 5.8

The reader is asked to respond to the 'felt experience' of three questions. Arguably this may not address the individuality of a person's dementia or the unique burden(s) this can have on a family/partner. What would you feel and think if:

- as a person with dementia – I am increasingly becoming reliant on other people for how I spend my waking days
- as an adult family member/partner – I live daily with the consequences of dementia and the restrictions this has on me and my lifestyle and choices
- as a family child/young person – I live with and witness the changes dementia has caused and the uncertainties the future will have for the person I know/knew.

Activity 5.8 conjures up *stage theories* of dementia, which measure *progress* in terms of ongoing deterioration. It is a theoretical position that was challenged by Tom Kitwood (1997) as failing to recognize the uniqueness of each person as well as their capacity for new growth or regaining functions thought to have been lost, something he termed *rementia*. Whilst this position is similarly challenged by a number of service-user advocates who are leading by example and strongly demonstrating their *living beyond dementia* (Swaffer 2016), there remains an enduring view of a person's decline as measured in stages of:

- mild
- moderate
- severe.

These stages appear in cognitive tests such as the MMSE with scores suggesting cognitive ability at various stages (Alzheimer's Association 2019). Therefore, it is unsurprising if measuring oneself against a descending line on a graph and projecting oneself into various points in the future that an individual is likely to be left with feelings of hopelessness and depression. This can be reinforced through an acknowledgement of losses that are occurring and their significance to those involved. Consider, for example, as mentioned above, how the gifted writer Iris Murdoch might have felt when faced with her dwindling ability in something core to her very sense of self – *words*. Similarly, another author with dementia, Terry Pratchett, in his Richard Dimbleby lecture, made an impassioned plea for euthanasia (*The Guardian* 2010). The BBC TV documentary *My Life on a Post It Note* (2006) featured Christine, a bright and bubbly woman trying to come to terms with her fading abilities and independence. She spoke about euthanasia or the contemplation of swimming out to sea and simply not returning. Lisa Genova's (2007) fictional novel *Still Alice* also covered this topic with the central character Alice, a cognitive psychology professor diagnosed with dementia, preparing a reminder to herself, and the means of taking her life should she reach a particular level of deficit. The fact that individuals are contemplating taking their lives as a consequence of their dementia experience illustrates the level of hopelessness and helplessness felt and consequently a need for support and sharing of fears and feelings.

Family carers

An issue concerns the lack of support and understanding from wider family members leaving the carer feeling very isolated within their role. The relentless nature of a family carer's role, coupled with this lack of opportunities to feel acknowledged and supported, can leave a person feeling anguished and despairing. Chris Carling (2012, p.138), caring for both parents with dementia, expressed: 'What I know about my own feelings is that they lie beneath a calm, coping surface, reluctant to declare themselves too much for fear of...what? Too much pain? Being overwhelmed by emotion?'

This impactful narrative shows the fear that one can have about the potency of one's own misery and distress and the inability to share or own one's feelings with the concern of overwhelming oneself or others. There is something poignant about helplessly observing another person' deterioration yet feeling unable to bring about any relief. The emotional impact on a family member who becomes the main carer is heightened through having to witness changes in the feelings, thoughts and behaviours of the person they have shared their life with. Feelings of gradually losing touch can evoke such severe consequences for both that they feel like they are living as strangers. The distress experienced by carers can be multi-faceted and include that of grief, prior to a person with dementia's death, in part because of the series of losses they experience and the chronic nature of caregiving (Mulligan 2012). Results from research with 202 spousal and adult child caregivers of people with dementia suggest that grief is a significant component of the caregiving experience, and is related to, but distinct from, depression. Lindauer and Harvath (2014) offer a definition of pre-death grief in dementia family members, where pre-death grief in the context of dementia family caregiving is the caregiver's emotional and physical response to the perceived losses in a valued recipient. They argue that family caregivers experience a variety of emotions that wax and wane over the course of a dementing disease. According to Blandin and Pepin (2015), dementia grief is distinguished from anticipatory grief by disruptions in communications and impairments in awareness that occur even early on in the disease. With most terminal medical conditions, there is an opportunity for conflict resolution and sharing feelings between the dying person and their family members up until death. This opportunity for similar resolution is limited for dementia caregivers due to language deficits and a lack of insight in the person receiving care resulting from disruptions in reasoning that can manifest themselves in the early stages of dementia.

For young people, the feelings and experiences in connection with witnessing a parent's gradual deterioration evoke much trepidation and anxiety for the future. Allen *et al.* (2009) studied the impact that a father's dementia had upon young people (aged 13–24 years), identifying five main themes of damage of dementia, recognition of relationships, strain, caring and coping.

* * *

The sense of despair and hopelessness will be compounded through the degree of discrimination experienced. *Our Dementia, Our Rights* (Hare 2016) provides evidence on the plight of many people with dementia and their families who have found it hard to get the services or support they need, or to know their entitlements. They have experienced treatment that can be regarded as contravening their human rights.

Another issue that will cause much unsettlement and upset especially when behaviour is in sharp contrast to previous experiences is that of abuse from the person with dementia. In the BBC documentary *Malcolm and Barbara*, Barbara can be heard repeatedly exclaiming 'You're hurting me' when grasped painfully by her hair or around the wrists. Her expressed sense of desperation is all the more striking given her assertion that prior to his diagnosis Malcolm was never violent towards her. Similarly, the documentary *The Trouble with Dad* with David Baddiel showcased a number of families where the aggression demonstrated by a person with Pick's disease dementia was in marked contrast to their earlier lives. It is difficult to imagine the feelings of desperation of family members through having to share their living space with someone who is becoming increasingly more a stranger to them as well as becoming more demanding and aggressive.

How true could this be today?

The theme of 'How true could this be today?' asks you to consider reframing an observation from the past. This commentary had an influence in informing thinking at that time whilst also determining opinions of the day. A number of questions will encourage you to consider its relevance in the here and now, such as: have national opinions changed or not? Do you agree or not with these comments? What has influenced your attitudes?

Background information: Lubinski (1991) proposed that learned behaviours may arise as a consequence of the perceptions or beliefs adopted by others and that 'learned helplessness' and a cycle of incompetence can be triggered by the diagnosis of dementia.

- Do you agree or not with this these observations from the 1990s?
- Do you think that a diagnosis of dementia, in present times, carries certain expectations such as learned helplessness for the individual?
- Can you identify other expectations that the public has towards individuals with a diagnosis of dementia?
- What evidence have you for the above responses?

Concluding thoughts

This chapter has a tenet of 'struggling' and covers some of the taxing and unendurable aspects that the dementia experience can entail. It has been concerned with central elements such as 'Who am I?' and fears of losing the essence of self. Isolation and despair have also been covered. The difficulty and pessimism reflected here represent, however, only one end of the spectrum. The opposite pole *coping* is more about optimism and is covered in the next chapter.

PERSONAL LEARNING

What was your past knowledge and understanding, what new learning have you achieved and how could this inform your future personal and/or professional interventions?

As a 'family member', my new learning includes ....

....

On reading the first-person narratives, my new learning includes

....

INTERVENTIONS

Be mindful that whatever comments are offered should be realistic, achievable and person-centred. Also, that the feelings conveyed and observations made reinforce the 'struggles experienced' for the individual and significant other people in their life.

The types of interventions could include ....

....

References

Allen, J., Oyebode, J.R. and Allen, J. (2009). 'Having a father with young onset dementia: the impact on well-being of young people.' *Dementia: The International Journal of Social Research and Practice 8* (4), 455–480.

Alzheimer's Association (2019). *Medical Tests.* Accessed on 1/12/19 at www.alz.org/alzheimers-dementia/diagnosis/medical_tests.

Alzheimer's Disease International (2019). *World Alzheimer Report 2019: Attitudes to Dementia.* London: Alzheimer's Disease International.

Alzheimer's Research UK (2015). *Dementia in the Family*. Cambridge: Alzheimer's Research UK.

Alzheimer's Society (2009). *Living with Dementia*. Accessed on 12/1/17 at www.alzheimers.org.uk.

Alzheimer's Society (2017). *ONS reports unpaid carers provide social care worth £57 billion, Alzheimer's Society comments*. Accessed on 7/8/18 at www.alzheimers.org.uk/news/2018-05-03/ons-reports-unpaid-carers-provide-social-care-worth-ps57-billion-alzheimers-society.

Archibald, C. (2003). 'Sexuality and dementia: the role dementia plays when expression becomes a component of residential care work.' *Alzheimer's Care Quarterly 4* (2), 37–48.

Batra, S., Sullivan, J. and Geldmacher, D. (2013). 'Qualitative assessment of self-identity in advanced dementia. Alzheimer's and Dementia.' Conference: Alzheimer's Association International Conference 2013. Boston, MA, US. Conference Publication, 9 (4), 643.

BBC (2006). *One Life: My Life on a Post It Note*. Accessed on 7/9/17 at https://forum.alzheimers.org.uk/threads/bbc-one-life-my-life-on-a-post-it-note.3357.

Beaumont, H. (2009). *Losing Clive to Younger Onset Dementia: One Family's Story*. London: Jessica Kingsley Publishers.

Behuniak, S. (2011). 'The living dead? The construction of people with Alzheimer's disease as zombies.' *Ageing and Society 31* (1), 70–92.

Benbow, S. and Jolley, D. (2012). 'Dementia: stigma and its effects.' *Neurodegenerative Disease Management 2* (2), 165.

Bender, M. and Cheston, R. (1997). 'Inhabitants of a lost kingdom: a model of the subjective experience of dementia.' *Ageing and Society 17* (5), 513–532.

Blandin, K. and Pepin, R. (2015). 'Dementia grief: a theoretical model of a unique grief experience.' *Dementia 16*, 67–78.

Bomford, A. and Doyle, E. (2019). 'Wanting to die at "five to midnight" – before dementia takes over.' 30 January. Accessed on 12/12/19 at www.bbc.co.uk/news/stories-47047579.

Bowlby, J. (1997). *Attachment*. London: Random House.

Brodaty, H. and Hadzi-Pavlovic, D. (2009). 'Psychosocial effects on carers of living with persons with dementia.' *Australian and New Zealand Journal of Psychiatry 24* (3), 351–361.

Bryden, C. (2018). *Will I Still Be Me? Finding a Continuing Sense of Self in the Lived Experience of Dementia*. London: Jessica Kingsley Publishers.

Cadell, L. and Clare, L. (2010). 'The impact of dementia on self and identity: a systematic review.' *Clinical Psychological Review 30* (1), 113–126.

Cahill S., O'Shea E. and Pierce M. (2012). *Creating Excellence in Dementia Care: A Research Review for Ireland's National Dementia Strategy*. Dublin: Trinity College Dublin.

Campbell P., Wright J., Oyebode J., Job, D., Crome, P., Bentham, P., Jones, L. and Lendon, C. (2008). 'Determinants of burden in those who care for someone with dementia.' *International Journal of Geriatric Psychiatry 23*, 1078–1085.

Carers UK (2010). *Carers Missing Millions: £840m of Carer's Allowance Goes Unclaimed*. Accessed on 24/1/20 at www.carersuk.org/news-and-campaigns/news/carers-missing-millions-840m-of-carer-s-allowance-goes-unclaimed.

Carers UK (2011). *Half a Million Voices: Improving Support for BAME Carers*. London: Carers UK.

Carers UK (2015). *Alarming Numbers of People Feel Isolated and Lonely as a Result of Caring for Their Loved Ones*. Accessed on 8/4/20 at www.carersuk.org/news-and-campaigns.

Carling, C. (2012). *But Then Something Happened*. Cambridge: Golden Books.

Channel 4 (2018). *Rainbow Café*. 21 April.

Channel 4 (2017). *The Trouble with Dad*. 20 February.

Clare, L. (2003). 'Managing threats to self: awareness in early stage Alzheimer's disease.' *Social Science and Medicine, 57* (6), 1017–1029.

Clark-McGhee, K. and Castro, M. (2015). 'A narrative analysis of poetry written from the words of people given a diagnosis of dementia.' *Dementia 14* (1), 9–26.

Davis, R. (1989). *My Journey into Alzheimer's Disease*. Bucks: Tyndale House Publishers.

Day, J., Anderson, R. and Davis, L. (2014). 'Compassion fatigue in adult daughter caregivers of a parent with dementia.' *Issues in Mental Health Nursing 35*, 796–804.

DeBaggio, T. (2002). *Losing My Mind: An Intimate Look at Alzheimer's*. New York: The Free Press.

Dewing, J. and Dijk, S. (2014). 'What is the current state of care for older people with dementia in general hospitals? A literature review.' *Dementia: International Journal of Social Research and Practice 15* (1), 106–124.

Dixey, R. (2016). *Our Dementia Diary: Irene, Alzheimer's and Me*. Surbiton: Medina Publishing Ltd.

Donnellan, W., Bennett, K. and Soulsby, L. (2017). 'Family close but friends closer: exploring social support and resilience in older spousal dementia carers.' *Aging and Mental Health 21* (11), 1222–1228.

Draper, B., Peisah, C., Snowdon, J. and Brodaty, H. (2010). 'Early dementia diagnosis and the risk of suicide and euthanasia.' *Alzheimer's and Dementia 6* (1), 75–82.

Duane, F., Brasher, K. and Koch, S. (2011). 'Living alone with dementia.' *Dementia 12 (1)*, 123–136.

Duggan, S., Blackman, T. and Martyr, A. (2008). 'The impact of early dementia on outdoor life: a "shrinking world"?' *Dementia 7* (2), 191–204.

Dupuis, S. (2002). 'Understanding ambiguous loss in the context of dementia care.' *Journal of Gerontological Social Work 37* (2), 93–115.

Ettema, T., Dröes, R., de Lange, J., Mellenbergh, G. and Ribbe, M. (2007). 'QUALIDEM: development and evaluation of a dementia specific quality of life instrument – validation.' *International Journal of Geriatric Psychiatry 22* (5), 424–430.

Fassio, M. (2009). *Dementia and Mum. Who Really Cares?* London: Kew Bridge Press.

Friel McGowin, D. (1994). *Living in the Labyrinth: A Personal Journey Through the Maze of Alzheimer's*. New York: Delta.

Genova, L. (2007). *Still Alice*. New York: Simon and Schuster.

Gillies, A. (2009). *Keeper: A Book about Memory, Identity, Isolation, Wordsworth and Cake*. London: Short Books.

Goffman, E. (1963). *Stigma*. New York: Simon and Schuster.

Guardian, The (2010). 'Terry Pratchett: my case for a euthanasia tribunal.' 1 February. Accessed on 15/8/14 at www.theguardian.com.

Haak, N. (2002). 'Maintaining connections: understanding communication from the perspective of persons with dementia.' *Alzheimer's Care Quarterly* 3 (2), 116–131.

Hare, P. (2016). *Our Dementia, Our Rights. DEEP*. Exeter: Innovations in Dementia.

Harrison, J. (2001). 'It's none of my business: gay and lesbian invisibility in aged care.' *Australian Occupational Therapy Journal 48* (3), 142–145.

Hart, B. and Wells, D. (1997). 'The effects of language used by caregivers on agitation in residents with dementia.' *Clinical Nurse Specialist 11* (1), 20–23.

Hawkley, L. and Cacioppo, J. (2010). 'Loneliness matters: a theoretical and empirical review of consequences and mechanisms.' *Annals of Behavioral Medicine 40*, 218–227.

Herrmann, L.K., Welter, E., Leverenz, J.B., Lerner, A., Udelson, N., Kanetsky, C. and Sajatovic, M. (2018). 'A systematic review of Alzheimer's disease and dementia stigma research: how might we move the stigma dial?' *American Journal of Geriatric Psychiatry 26* (3), 316–331.

Holt, I., and Morris, G. (2015). *Leading nurses to guide health role transition from a metasynthesis of dementia literature*. Sigma Theta Tau: Phi Mu Chapter Biannual Conference. Weetwood Hall Conference Centre, Leeds.

Hutchinson, K., Roberts, R., Daly, M. and Bulsara, M. (2016). 'Empowerment of young people who have a parent living with dementia: a social model perspective.' *International Psychogeriatrics 28* (4), 657–668.

ITV1 (2007). *Malcolm and Barbara*. 8 August.

Joinson, A. (1992). 'Coping with compassion fatigue.' *Nursing 2* (4), 116–122.

Kitwood, T. (1997). *Dementia Reconsidered*. Maidenhead: Open University Press.

Kozberg, C. (n.d.). *A Jewish Response to Dementia: Honoring Broken Tablets*. Accessed on 15/12/19 at www.caregiverslibrary.org/portals/0/Microsoft%20Word%20-%20A%20Jewish%20Response%20to%20Dementia[1].pdf.

Lee, D., McKeith, I., Mosimann, U., Ghosh-Nodyal, A. and Thomas, A. (2013). 'Examining carer stress in dementia: the role of subtype diagnosis and neuropsychiatric symptoms.' *International Journal of Geriatric Psychiatry 28* (2), 135–141.

Lindauer, A. and Harvath, T. (2014). 'Pre-death grief in the context of dementia caregiving: a concept analysis.' *Journal of Advanced Nursing 70* (10), 2196–2207.

Link, B. and Phelan, J. (2001). 'Conceptualizing stigma.' *Annual Review of Sociology 27*, 363–385.

Lowery, K., Mynt, P., Aisbett, J., Dixon, T., O'Brien, J. and Ballard, C. (2000). 'Depression in the carers of dementia sufferers: a comparison of the carers of patients suffering from dementia with Lewy bodies and the carers of patients with Alzheimer's disease.' *Journal of Affective Disorders 59*, 61–65.

Lubinski, R. (1991). *Dementia and Communication*. Philadelphia, PA: B.C. Decker.

Mace, N. and Rabins, R. (2012). *The 36-Hour Day: A Family Guide to Caring for People Who Have Alzheimer's Disease, Related Dementias, and Memory Loss (5th Edition).* Baltimore: Johns Hopkins Press.

Mackenzie, J. (2006). 'Stigma and dementia: East European and South Asian family carers negotiating stigma in the UK.' *Dementia* 5, 233–247.

MDYB (2018). *Parents Caring for Adult Children with Dementia.* Accessed on 18/1/19 at https://makedementiayourbitch.com.

Memory Bridge (2009). *Gladys Wilson and Naomi Feil.* Accessed on 14/5/15 at www.youtube.com.

Merriman, R. (2015). 'TV Presenter Fiona Phillips opens up about how Alzheimer's changed her life and why she fears "disappearing".' Accessed on 6/9/17 at www.mirror.co.uk/3am/celebrity-news/tv-presenter-fiona-phillips-opens-6369014.

Milne, A. (2010). 'The "D" word: reflections on the relationship between stigma, discrimination and dementia.' *Journal of Mental Health, 19* (3), 227–233.

Mitchell, G., Dupuis, S. and Kontos, P. (2013). 'Dementia discourse: from imposed suffering to knowing other-wise.' *Journal of Applied Hermeneutics 12* (5), 1–19.

Mitchell, W. (2018). *Somebody I Used to Know.* London: Bloomsbury Publishing.

Mitchell, W. (2019). *Woman's Hour.* Accessed on 25/10/19 at www.bbc.co.uk/programmes/m000356z.

Moriarty, J., Sharif, N. and Robinson, J. (2011). 'Black and minority ethnic people with dementia and their access to support and services.' Accessed on 16/5/17 at https://kclpure.kcl.ac.uk/portal/files/13501330/SCIE_briefing.pdf.

Moyle, W., Kellett, U. and Ballantyne, A. (2011). 'Dementia and loneliness: an Australian perspective.' *Journal of Clinical Nursing 20* (9–10), 1445–1453.

Mulligan, E. (2012). 'Grief among dementia caregivers: a comparison of two assessment systems.' *Dissertation Abstracts International: Section B: The Sciences and Engineering 72* (12-B), 7693.

National Children's Bureau (2016). *Young People Caring for Adults with Dementia in England.* Accessed on 2/10/18 at www.ncb.org.uk/sites/default/files/field/attachment/news/young_people_caring_for_adults_with_dementia.pdf.

Nazarko, L. (2009). 'Understanding dementia: diagnosis and development.' *British Journal of Healthcare Assistants 5* (5), 216–220.

Nebes, R. and Brady, C. (1992). 'Generalized cognitive slowing and severity of dementia in Alzheimer's disease: implications for the interpretation of response-time data.' *Journal of Clinical and Experimental Neuropsychology. 14* (2), 317–326.

Nehemas, A. (1999). 'Never further than dinner or tea.' *London Review of Books 21* (5.4), 16–17. Accessed on 18/6/20 at https://www.lrb.co.uk/the-paper/v21/n05/alexander-nehamas/never-further-than-dinner-or-tea.

Open University (2015). *Rene Descartes – 'I think, therefore I am'.* Accessed on 18/6/19 at www.open.edu.

Pakenham, K.I., Chiu, J., Bursnall, S., Cannon, T. and Okochi, M. (2006). 'The psychosocial impact of care giving on young people who have a parent with an illness or disability: comparisons between young caregivers and no caregivers.' *Rehabilitation Psychology 51* (2), 113–126.

Parveen, S., Peltier, C. and Oyebode J. (2017). 'Perceptions of dementia and use of services in minority ethnic communities: a scoping exercise.' *Health and Social Care in the Community 25*, 734–742.

Pearce, A., Clare, L. and Pistrang, N. (2002). 'Managing sense of self: coping in the early stages of Alzheimer's disease.' *Dementia 1* (2), 173–192.

Price, E. (2010). 'Coming out to care: gay and lesbian carers' experiences of dementia services.' *Health and Social Care 18* (2), 160–168.

Purandare, N., Oude Voshaar, R., Rodway, C., Bickley, H., Burns, A. and Kapur, N. (2009). 'Suicide in dementia: 9 year national clinical survey in England.' *British Journal of Psychiatry 194* (2), 175–180.

Ryle, A. (1997). *Cognitive Analytic Therapy: Active Participation in Change.* Chichester: John Wiley and Sons.

Sabat, S. and Harré, R. (1992). 'The construction and deconstruction of self in Alzheimer's disease.' *Ageing and Society. 12* (4), 443–461.

Shenk, D. (2003). *The Forgetting: Alzheimer's: Portrait of an Epidemic.* New York: Anchor Books.

Sikes, P. (2017). *Perceptions and Experiences of Children and Young People with a Parent with Dementia.* Accessed on 9/10/19 at www.alzheimers.org.uk/research/our-research/research-projects/perceptions-experiences-children-young-people-parent-dementia.

Sikes, P. and Hall, M. (2016). 'It was then that I thought "whaat? This is not my Dad": the implications of the "still the same person" narrative for children and young people who have a parent with dementia.' *Dementia 17* (2), 180–198.

Sikes, P. and Hall, M. (2017). '"Every time I see him he's the worst he's ever been and the best he'll ever be": grief and sadness in children and young people who have a parent with dementia.' *Mortality 22* (4), 324–338.

Stephens, S., Kenny, R., Rowan, E., Allan. L., Kalaria, R., Bradbury, M. and Ballard, C. (2004). 'Neuropsychological characteristics of mild vascular cognitive impairment and dementia after stroke.' *International Journal of Geriatric Psychiatry 19* (11), 1053–1057.

Sutton, L. (2003). 'When late life brings a diagnosis of Alzheimer's disease and early life brought trauma. A cognitive-analytic understanding of loss of mind.' *Psychological Therapy with Older Adults 10* (3), 156–164.

Svanberg, E., Stott, J. and Spector A. (2010). '"Just helping": children living with a parent with young onset dementia.' *Aging and Mental Health 14* (6), 740–751.

Swaffer, K. (2013a). *Alone in a Crowd*. Accessed on 23/6/20 at https://kateswaffer.com/2013/11/02/alone-in-a-crowd.

Swaffer, K. (2013b). *Saturday Poem: Alone*. Accessed on 23/6/20 at https://kateswaffer.com/2013/07/13/saturday-poem-alone.

Swaffer, K. (2016). *What the Hell Happened to My Brain? Living Beyond Dementia*. London: Jessica Kingsley Publishers.

Swaffer, K. (n.d.). *The Impact on Parents and Partners*. Accessed on 18/6/19 at www.youngdementiauk.org/impact-parents-partners.

Talbot, M. (2011). *Keeping Mum: Caring for Someone with Dementia*. London: Hay House.

Telegraph, The (2013). 'Dementia couple: "Our world is shrinking".' 11 December. Accessed on 18/11/18 at www.telegraph.co.uk/news/health/elder/10511110/Dementia-couple-Our-world-is-shrinking.html.

Ward, R., Vass, A., Aggarwal, N., Garfield, C. and Cybyk, B. (2005). 'A kiss is still a kiss? The construction of sexuality in dementia care.' *Dementia 4* (1), 49–72.

Weiss, R. (1973). *Loneliness: The Experience of Emotional and Social Isolation*. Cambridge: MIT Press.

Yorkshire Evening Post (2013). 'Hidden army of Leeds carers is missing out on millions.' Accessed on 1/5/19 at www.yorkshireeveningpost.co.uk.

Zhu, C., Scarmeas, N., Ornstein, K., Albert, M., Brandt, J., Blacker, D., Sano, M. and Stern, Y. (2015). 'Health-care use and cost in dementia caregivers: longitudinal results from the Predictors Caregiver Study.' *Alzheimer's and Dementia 11* (4), 444–454.

Part 3

Living Beyond Dementia

Chapter 6

Coping

Introduction

The previous chapter addressed some of the difficulties and travails experienced by those with dementia and their families, focusing primarily upon the perspective of *struggling*. This perhaps fits more with common assumptions and expectations of the dementia experience with the concept of a person as a *dementia sufferer*. Whilst severe difficulties and distress are clearly encountered it does not define the totality of the dementia experience, which can be seen as existing as a movable point on a continuum between *struggling* and *coping*. This chapter is concerned with the opposing pole of *coping*, covering some of the ways that people with dementia continue to live well and experience quality of life.

The IDEAL study, a five-year longitudinal cohort study of the experiences of 1500 people with dementia and their family carers across Great Britain, aims to determine how social and psychological circumstances and available resources influence the ability to live well with dementia (Clare *et al.* 2014). It also seeks to identify what can be done by individuals, communities, health and social care practitioners, care providers and policy-makers to improve the likelihood of living well with dementia. The importance of well-being and coping within dementia is also emphasized by the National Dementia Strategy (Department of Health and Social Care 2009). This advocates an agenda of hope, stressing and validating the importance of the person who remains despite the presence of dementia. It encourages approaches for living well with dementia and provides a viable option to complement research initiatives searching for medical breakthroughs. With the right support, environmental adjustments, appropriate interventions and opportunities, people with dementia and their families can continue not only to live well but also to achieve new learning, remain productive, provide support for others and enjoy success with a variety of goals and targets.

The story so far

The Lawrence family have begun contemplating how their lives are being affected through the changes taking place. The start of their collective dementia journey has involved significant role transitions and is placing strain upon familial relationships. Each member has their own particular set of burdens to negotiate along with a growing sense of separateness and isolation. They are also having to contend with what is seen as Peter's loss of self as well as the threats to their identities as a couple or as a family. The difficulties are causing extreme distress and engendering feelings of despair.

Chapter themes

This chapter will introduce the reader to the following themes:

- Living beyond dementia – 'I'm still here'
- Peer support – 'I'm not alone'
- Creative arts (self-expression and therapeutic benefits) – 'Finding my voice'

The themes identified here consider the *person* who continues to function post-diagnosis. The notion of *living beyond dementia* as advocated by Kate Swaffer (2016) provides a direct challenge to the restrictive pessimism often associated with this condition. This emphasizes the person who is 'still here' and with a life still to live alongside their dementia. The growing feelings of isolation and separateness that commonly occur for those with dementia and their families are addressed by examining peer support, an arena offering huge value to all parties in fostering a sense of engagement and mutual giving and receiving of support. Finally, the potency of the creative arts for those affected by dementia will be reviewed. This includes approaches and interventions that facilitate self-expression and provide individuals with a means of communication when words start to disappear. Collectively, the elements to be covered in this chapter examine some potent means by which coping and living well within the dementia experience are promoted and facilitated.

Living beyond dementia ('I'm still here')

This section deals with positivity, recognizing life as continuing post-diagnosis. It directly challenges the commonly applied and accepted negative assumptions where individuals and their families view the future in terms of impending restrictions and losses. This pessimistic framework regards dementia predominantly in terms of what can be considered *stages of decline* with individuals progressing steadily through 'mild' (early) and 'moderate' (middle) stages before reaching the 'severe' (late-stage) categorization. It is a reductionist view that is challenged by Kitwood (1997) as ill-defining the totality of the dementia experience. The focus upon declining abilities and functions not surprisingly evokes apprehension in relation to the future and can subsequently influence restrictive approaches and responses. The following section is focused specifically upon contrasting perspectives acknowledging the functions and abilities that people retain, and, importantly, new ones which they can develop.

Gill's Narrative 6.1: 'We have much to offer'

'Why is it that people get so preoccupied with the things that those with dementia can't do anymore or aspects they struggle with? I have now had plenty of opportunities to challenge my own thinking about this, especially given some of the new activities Peter and I are now involved with. We have both become ambassadors for the Alzheimer's Society, helping others to gain better understanding about the experience of living with dementia. We are just back from a conference in London, which both Peter and I gave a short presentation to. It was very nerve-wracking but very reassuring to meet other presenters who are going through similar experiences and who we felt we could strongly relate to. A further and very welcome benefit is the fact that we have something we are both involved with, which, as well as feeling productive, helps us feel more "husband and wife" than "person with dementia and carer".

I have also noticed that as Peter's confidence has grown he is involving himself again in activities he stopped doing some months ago. It is so nice to see him going out cycling with Tom. He has also signed up for an evening class in pottery, which he seems to enjoy. I do notice he is much calmer and less agitated when he returns home.'

- *Do you agree or not with Gill's optimism?*
- *What do you think Gill could gain from their involvement with local community groups, or what benefits could these give to her?*

Gill's narrative places a firm focus upon the life that she and her husband Peter are continuing to live. It also reaffirms their continued status as a couple, sharing in activities and acting in partnership with each other. Peter's continued productivity is a core aspect here, which opposes the predominance often given to loss and slowly deteriorating abilities. Here we have the sense of individuals involving themselves in new activities, which provides a stark contrast to the representation of change by a steadily declining line on a graph. The focus upon new learning, allied with attending to the skills and abilities individuals retain, will naturally seem a lot more encouraging and foster better opportunities for well-being. We can also consider the potential for regaining faculties and abilities presumed lost through one's deteriorating cognition as encapsulated through Kitwood's (1997) concept of *rementia*. This questions the extent to which declining functions are caused solely through organic changes taking place in the structure of the brain. Instead, psycho-social factors can be considered and confronted head on. For example, co-existing depression and anxiety will impede daily functioning with resultant symptoms easily confused with symptoms relating to a person's dementia. Likewise, environmental considerations or the attitudes of others can pose restrictions and lower a person's confidence and self-autonomy.

Essentially, this section challenges the predominance placed upon problems and difficulties, something that Swinton (2012) refers to as 'defectology'. Michael Ignatieff's fictional account *Scar Tissue* (1993) provides a strong illustration of how a person and their capabilities can be framed very differently in relation to the views and attitudes held by others. In his text, one brother continued to strongly appreciate his mother for who she was, despite her experience of dementia, whilst the other mainly acknowledged and saw what was being lost. These perspectives had a potent impact upon the quality of the relationship each continued to have with their mother. Gill and Peter's experience, whilst maybe not transferable to all affected by dementia, speaks about continued productivity. In this case it reflects what increasing numbers of people with dementia are doing: acting as advocates and sharing their personal narratives across a range of public forums. Speaking at conferences or relating personal experiences through blogs, discussion forums, workshops or other means provide vital opportunities for awareness-raising by people who can rightly be called *experts by experience* (Morris 2017). The benefits are also felt by those participating in terms of having their continued worth validated and appreciated by others.

Figure 6.1 considers attitudinal and behavioural dynamics that can promote the person as remaining central to their environment (family, friends and others) rather than their diagnosis dominating their life. However, if their coping approaches, degree of acceptance and responses and abilities become discouraged, the consequences could engender a reversal where dementia symptoms prevail in the person's interactions with their environment.

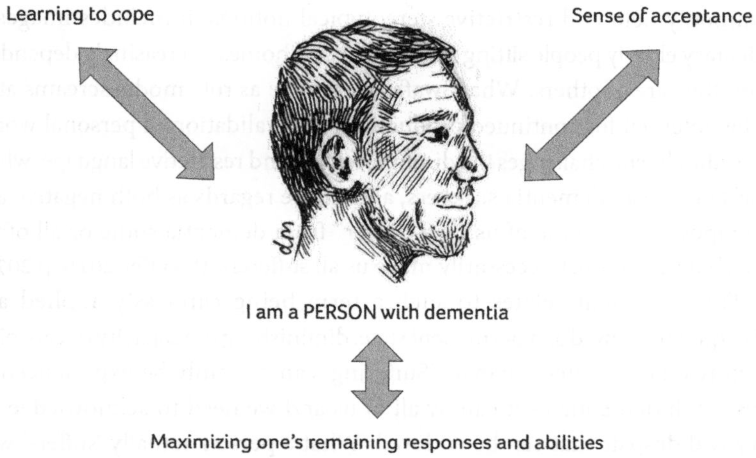

Figure 6.1 The person within

Kate Swaffer, a prominent campaigner and advocate, was diagnosed with dementia at the age of 49. She is a powerful role model, passionately involved in challenging negative and restrictive views towards those with dementia. As mentioned above, a core element within her advocacy work is the concept of *living beyond dementia*, a viewpoint that firmly emphasizes the life that individuals still have to live as well as their continued productivity (Swaffer 2014). She herself is testament to the notion of living beyond dementia, leading powerfully by example. This includes challenging what she terms Prescribed Disengagement®, an attitudinal position that engenders lowered attitudes towards those with dementia. She has rightly received many honours for her campaigning work, having authored a number of articles and books, completing Bachelor's and Master's degrees and holding membership of many bodies and organizations, all following her dementia diagnosis (Swaffer 2016). As if this wasn't enough, and what to some might seem astonishing, is her commencement of PhD study (Swaffer 2018). Whilst her achievements may not necessarily be replicable by others with dementia they do indeed serve as an inspiration, prompting others to strive towards what they might set as their own personal goals as well as opposing restrictive attitudes, either externally or internally driven. The challenge relating to attitudes was expressively articulated by Iain McGregor (Director of Spring Mount Nursing Home in Bradford, UK) who worked closely with Tom Kitwood: 'Dementia can be regarded as a product of our low expectations' (Link 1993).

This statement articulates how restrictions can be internally or externally applied with the championing of living beyond dementia serving to challenge commonly held and restrictive stereotypical notions. It includes images of sedentary elderly people sitting passively in care homes, increasingly dependent upon the care of others. What Swaffer's example as role model screams at us is the potential for continued productivity and validation of personal worth. Accordingly, she challenges the disempowering and restrictive language, which labels people as 'dementia sufferers', a term she regards as both negative and disempowering: 'Some of us may "suffer" from dementia some or all of the time, but that doesn't necessarily make us all sufferers' (Swaffer 2016, p.207).

This comment relates to such a term being carelessly applied and subsequently viewed as a permanent state, diminishing the capacity or capability of individuals to affect change. 'Suffering' can certainly be experienced by those with dementia as it can by all of us and we need to acknowledge the very real despair that can be endured. What a person actually 'suffers' with or from, however, needn't be necessarily directly related to one's changing cognitive state or the bio-chemical and organic processes taking place in one's brain structure. Instead, we might consider the impact from lowered societal expectations, stigmatizing attitudes, increasing isolation and a pervading sense of hopelessness. Swaffer's example prompts us to rethink *dementia* and pursue the elements that facilitate the living of more productive lives.

ACTIVITY 6.1

Are you comfortable with the term 'dementia sufferer' and why?

Are your responses based upon personal and/or professional experiences?

A fellow Australian, Christine Bryden, former biochemist and subsequent dementia champion and advocate, also challenges attitudes towards people with dementia. These, she reflects, can often be patronizing and lacking in understanding of a person's daily battles (Bryden 2015). Her personal stance is very much that of survivor and is complemented by the optimistic message of: 'Enjoy each moment to the full!'

The longevity and breadth of her advocacy and campaigning work is highly impressive especially as it spans more than two decades (Bryden 2015). Her recent publication *Will I Still Be Me*? retains Kitwood's (1997) notion of personhood and focuses upon the internal journey experienced by those with dementia (Bryden 2018). This stresses how a continuing sense of self is possible post-diagnosis and contradicts the 'fading away' notion with individuals eventually becoming an 'empty shell'. It highlights something of the person who *still* exists and continues to have a life to live. This is reflected within Lisa Genova's (2007) potent fictional account *Still Alice* about psychology professor Alice Howland, who seeks to maintain her contributions to and involvement with society, as mentioned above.

Bryden (2018) challenges negative views of dementia and addresses the potential for individuals to live meaningfully with dementia. She identifies core elements of self as:

- *embodied self* – an aspect of my *self* that gives me my sense of being embodied as an 'I' with first-person feelings about the world around me, distinguishing self from non-self
- *rational self* – an aspect of my *self* that gives me my sense of being an embodied self in relationships with others, and with what gives me meaning
- *narrative self* – an aspect of my *self* that is able to find meaning in life and to develop a sense of narrative identity in the present moment.

This very eloquently expresses the continued sense of self that exists alongside a person's developing symptoms of dementia.

ACTIVITY 6.2

From your professional experience, if appropriate, what types of communication approaches would you consider using to encourage/ maintain a coping attitude? You may wish to place your responses in the following sub-groups:

- **visually (my body language and how I would present myself)**
- **verbally (the words I would use and check for understanding)**
- **vocally (my intonation and the ways I speak).**

British campaigner Wendy Mitchell's (2018) narrative *Somebody I Used to Know* presents a very eloquent and informative account of coping with dementia and continuing to live her life. Her narrative is endearing and thought-provoking, very much informing readers about the person behind the words, with her love of the restorative and refreshing properties of a good cup of tea coming across very clearly. She acts as an advocate and champion for the Alzheimer's Society maintaining an illuminating blog entitled 'Which Me Am I Today?' She previously worked as an NHS administrator, later bringing her organizational abilities to her role as dementia advocate. The information within her book's cover notes states: 'Wendy's journey as her dementia worsens is told with so little self-pity, so much humour, and so much insight. She counters the stereotypes of the media and the medical profession, and reminds us how much is possible, even with this cruel disease.'

This is poignantly striking and does indeed promote what 'is possible', rather than what might now be regarded as no longer attainable. Her text stands testament as a guide and model to promote positivity and hope within the dementia experience. Further feedback evidenced amongst Amazon's customers and the Alzheimer's Society Talking Point forum show how inspirational and helpful her work is to others living with dementia. What such championing of dementia does is to raise awareness as well as encouraging and inspiring others to continue with areas of productivity and importance within their lives. Indeed the sense of continuity of one's life and optimism is strongly promoted: 'It's worth remembering…that even as our memories fade, it's not too late for new ones to be made' (Mitchell 2018, p.232).

The concept of 'new memories' being created is a powerful one. These can indeed bring fulfilling and life-affirming experiences.

Nigel Hullah, former human rights lawyer diagnosed with posterior cortical atrophy, subsequently became a member of the Three Nations Dementia Working Group (England, Wales and Northern Ireland) and Dementia Engagement and Empowerment Project. His campaigning work on behalf of those with dementia urged them to have their say and be acknowledged for who they are, which he stressed was crucially needed as: 'Everybody saw me through the prism of dementia – I stopped being a person.'

He challenged this personally through his advocacy work showcasing the *person* that individuals like himself continue to be at all stages post-diagnosis (Alzheimer's Society 2018a). Likewise, another prominent campaigner, Helga Rohra (2016), self-proclaimed *dementia activist* and diagnosed with dementia with Lewy bodies, writes expressively and humorously about her 'battles' with bureaucrats and the technological systems that have replaced people with machines. Rohra also relates her election to the board of the Munich Alzheimer's Society as causing a stir of interest across Germany as their first member diagnosed with dementia. Her direct challenge to a *Süddeutsche Zeitung* (South German newspaper) photographer over his request to picture her sitting passively, instead requesting a more dynamic image of her next to an Alzheimer's Society poster, was telling of the impression she was determined to convey. Her vitality and articulateness were at odds with what might have been expected of someone with dementia, and she relates having to respond to people challenging her about the authenticity of her dementia diagnosis.

As with Christine Bryden (2005), who quietened dissenting conference delegates with images of her own brain scan, Rohra felt called upon to provide conclusive evidence that someone as expressive and able as her could indeed have dementia. In this instance though what is striking to note is that her *accuser* was a healthcare practitioner. The core message being transmitted by such role models as those featured above is that people with dementia can be articulate, successful, productive and independent. We need to question here the extent to which we might obstruct such aspects through a negative framing of dementia as a 'product of our low expectations'. Such 'lowered expectations' will be keenly felt in the workplace as related by Doug Banks, diagnosed in his fifties with posterior cortical atrophy. Although feeling able to continue working with some modifications in place, the response he met from prospective employers was less than welcoming and understanding (BBC 2019). As mentioned above, the Channel 4 programme *The Restaurant That Makes Mistakes* showcased a timely experiment involving a group of people with dementia taking over the running of a restaurant. As commented by one of the participants: 'It was exhausting, emotional, hilarious, fun and heart-breaking at times. But my overriding feeling is what fun we had' (*Dementia Together* 2019).

What was also notable was the improvement in cognitive function for a number of those taking part along with enhancements in self-confidence and self-esteem, feeling less isolated and disengaged and having a renewed sense of productivity. Essentially, this championed inclusivity, showing the very real value that individuals with multiple life experiences and occupational skills could still offer to the work setting.

ACTIVITY 6.3

Do you think organizations, for example, banks, supermarkets or government departments, have sufficiently promoted awareness and introduced technologies to meet the needs of a person with dementia?

If so, what have you observed?

If not, what do you think could be introduced?

The role models promoted in this section show people with dementia continuing to function and be recognized for their continued productivity. Such considerations need to extend to couples and families, seeing how they continue to operate as a partnership or collaborative unit even with dementia in their midst. The support of relevant parties can be core here as shown within Bryden's and Swaffer's narratives. In Kate Swaffer's (2019, p.240) case her husband is regarded by her as her BUB (Back-Up Brain):

> We think of a back-up brain as being the same as the hard drive in a computer. He said recently, it empowers him to be by my side and with me, rather than to 'care' for me, a very subtle but significant difference.

This expresses the ability for them to continue side by side as partners as opposed to carer and cared for. The retention of former familial roles importantly helps to maintain relationships. Wendy Mitchell's daughter Sarah was interviewed in Radio 4's *Woman's Hour* (BBC 2019) and related her pride regarding her mother's continued independence and achievements. The need to recognize and support independence, though, is not without difficulty as: 'When she's struggling I want to intrude and it might make me feel better though would make mum feel worse.'

She also relates how much closer the family have become and the deeper level at which they now converse with each other. Essentially, their relationship remains very much as 'daughter and mother' as opposed to 'carer and carer for'.

Interventions aimed at supporting family members with their continued lives include the provision of individual sessions. Selwood *et al.* (2007) found excellent evidence for the efficacy of six or more sessions of individual behavioural management therapy for teaching caregivers coping strategies. Examples of individual work include the Early Diagnosis Dyadic Intervention

Programme, which provides structured, time-limited individual counselling for family caregivers and care receivers in the early stages of dementia (Whitlatch *et al.* 2006). Findings outlined the value in engaging in dialogue about future preferences for care and related uncertainty and worries.

This section featured discussion around the theme 'Living beyond dementia', which importantly outlines the continued lives of all family members. The concept 'I'm still here' provides a potent counter to the pessimism commonly felt. This not only applies to the person with dementia but can be encapsulated as relating to partners – 'We are still a couple' and children – 'We are still a family' or, for example, 'He is still my father'. The term 'still' therefore promotes continuation and normalcy, which are key in helping individuals traverse and face with confidence the related changes taking place.

> **EXERCISE:** IN SEARCH OF 'DEMENTIA FRIENDLINESS'
>
> This exercise asks you to explore personal thoughts, feelings and possible behaviours on the theme of 'dementia friendliness' by exploring community provision. (See Chapter 8.)

Peer support ('I am not alone')

People with dementia and their carers express the importance of having connection with others who are in a similar situation. One of Yalom's (2005) identified curative factors within therapeutic groups is that of *universality*, denoting the concept 'I am not alone'. This is a very potent and striking element noting the sense of connectedness felt with others and a means of receiving validation of one's own experience. Indeed, the Alzheimer's Café UK have adopted the logo and slogan 'All in the same boat'. For people with dementia and their families, peer support can provide a lifeline helping to combat the growing sense of separateness, difference and isolation. This is where engaging with peers, those with relatable experience, has immense value to offer. It is especially important for groups such as those with young-onset dementia or from within the LGBT community who often feel overlooked by dementia services. Specific approaches targeting these groups such as the setting up of the LGBT Dementia Support Network have proved invaluable (Newman and Price 2012).

In unpicking what peer support actually relates to we are met with a wide variety of resources and innovations providing support and guidance for people with dementia and their families. This includes face-to-face meetings through activity groups and dementia cafés, but much can also be found within the growing set of internet resources. The focus upon the online community will address two particular resource types, namely blogs and discussion forums.

Gill's Narrative 6.2: Feeling connected

'I cannot sing the praises enough of the wonderful people we have met over the last year. Meeting others in a similar position to us has been inspiring and immensely consoling. We are friends now with a number of individuals and couples who truly understand and "get" what we are going through. These are people who genuinely accept us for who we are and importantly are not fazed by the spectre of dementia. Our social life has been restored and we regularly meet up with them not only through organized events but also more casually for coffee or maybe a meal. These wonderful people have given us back a feeling of "normality", which I thought was lost. It has also been great for the family. Ashleigh and Tom (and even little Hannah) have attended some of the activities at the day centre and seemed to enjoy their time there.

Peter has commenced his own blog detailing our daily experiences. This has really taken off. He asked me to add some of my thoughts and it has gradually developed into a shared blog, which I am told is a bit of a first and fairly unique. We have had some very positive and heart-affirming responses from those reading our posts.'

- *Do you think there could be any benefits for Gill and Peter in 'publishing' their daily life experiences?*
- *Can blogging sites offer a person's felt experiences of their dementia?*

Gill's narrative expressed some very powerful elements including the notion of feeling connected with and understood by others, people who are importantly not 'fazed' by dementia. Another element that resonates strongly is the sense of 'normality' that is restored to the family through these approaches and the value of this cannot be underestimated. Consider for a moment what this means to families who have perhaps previously experienced increasing feelings of difference and alienation from their everyday lives. Here, within their redeveloped social worlds, they can find acceptance, solace and friendship. There is a strong degree of hope and optimism expressed within Gill's words showing the sense of autonomy being embraced by those with dementia and their families, who are taking charge of their lives. The focus within this section will in turn address the perspectives of:

- the person with dementia
- carers and family members.

Person with dementia

Willis, Semple and de Waal's (2018) study examined three dementia peer support groups in South London. Key outcomes noted for people with dementia were mental stimulation and a reduction in loneliness and isolation. Theurer and Hall (2016) found peer support to be positively associated with well-being, showing a decrease in the rate of physical decline, loneliness and depression. Their study highlighted that participating in a peer support group benefits those with dementia, offering emotional and practical support, as well as increasing self-esteem through the opportunities to help others. One group participant notably commented: 'It takes the loneliness away.'

As outlined by the Health Innovation Network (2015), peer support for people with dementia:

- improves well-being through improved social and emotional support as a result of shared experiences and building of new social networks
- reduces loneliness (people with dementia frequently report feeling excluded and isolated)
- improves physical health through practical support, such as medication reminders and general information about staying healthy.

The key elements shown here are concerned with feeling engaged and connected with like-minded people, lessening isolation and supporting well-being. As addressed above, peer support provides important opportunities to meet others and share experiences with those who are regarded as being in a similar situation. This type of support, though, is not available in all localities and in some areas can be oversubscribed or difficult to access. The younger age onset group in particular are poorly supported by the resources that are available (Rabanal *et al.* 2018) and there is little that is culturally specific for black and minority ethnic groups (Moriarty, Sharif and Robinson 2011). The following narrative of a person with dementia from the Health Innovation Network (2015) expresses an essential function provided by peer support for those living with dementia:

> When you have dementia, you're fighting with yourself all the time – it is hard work! You're struggling all the time to be what you'd call 'normal' but coming here is safe and relaxing. I can be myself here because I'm not worried about saying the wrong thing. (Health Innovation Network 2015)

Certain words stand out here in stark detail such as 'normal', 'safe' and 'relaxing'. To start with, the importance of enhancing and reconnecting individuals with feeling 'normal' reflects sentiments expressed in Gill's narrative of finding it hard being regarded as different. As featured in Chapter 4, the start of a person's journey with dementia can be marked by a perceived distinction from their former pre-diagnostic state of being a person *without a condition*. Having dementia can change how the sense of self is viewed and engender expectations in terms of how one might be treated and regarded by others. Therefore, meeting peers can feel like a breath of fresh air, enhancing one's sense of normality through being related to more as a person than a condition. The next words 'safe' and 'relaxing' show a powerful function through innovations and environments where individuals can feel secure. This is significant given the degree to which people might feel increasingly uncertain and tense. The narrative above reflects the feeling of freedom to be oneself, to be accepted for who one is in the present as well as having one's difficulties unconditionally accepted. This type of support can also enable people to feel that they can continue to live well, even with dementia, as the following narrative expresses: 'To date old friendships have been renewed, interests and hobbies restarted, new activities begun and friendships developed, both via peer support groups and through accessing other groups and activities' (Health Innovation Network 2015).

As well as stressing what is maintained or restarted from one's life this narrative also includes the word 'new' in relation to activities and friendships. This reflects Swaffer's (2016) concept of *living beyond dementia*, denoting the life that is still to be lived following one's diagnosis.

Nigel Hullah's *life-saving* experience of peer support from the Swansea-based group Fuse and Muse is shared in the Alzheimer's Society's *Dementia Together* magazine (2019):

> Sometimes dementia whispers in my ear, 'Nigel, you ain't strong enough to withstand the storm.' But one phone call, conversation or meeting with my group and I'm able to say to dementia, 'I am the storm.' There is no support like peer support – it has saved my life.

This forceful message shouts at us the need to consider initiatives such as these and the invaluable potential peer support has for those with dementia.

Carers and family members

The sense of connectedness felt by those with dementia from peer support can be extended to encompass carers and family members regarding contact with those who might be described as fellow travellers. Marianne Talbot (2011, p.13) describes attending a carer's workshop as both eye-opening and heart-rending. She did, though, find it cheering being able to share stories with people in the same position, and especially remarked upon the wry humour found in sharing difficult and stressful situations: 'There are plenty of tears, a pall of anxiety, and manifest exhaustion. But the odd thing is that it very quickly becomes funny.'

This laughter here is evidently not an avoidance of the very real distress and hardship felt but more a needed release of emotions in the safety and companionship of people who 'get it'. Indeed, Willis, Semple and de Waal (2018) show peer support groups as helping to reduce stress and the perceived burden of care. Lauritzen *et al.*'s (2015) study found that peer support provided a source of positive emotional support and a means of venting negative feeling and gaining help to address issues in the everyday life of caring for older adults with dementia. This is supported by Smith *et al.*'s (2018) qualitative findings, which show peer support to be an important source of emotional and social support for carers. According to Keyes *et al.* (2016), peer support had positive emotional and social impact grounded in the identification with others, noting commonality of experience and reciprocity of support. Participants also felt more acknowledged and helped by support received by peers as opposed to healthcare professionals. The key message being relayed here is that of truly feeling heard and understood.

An issue perhaps to consider is how closely it is perceived that others relate to one's experiences, which can influence the degree of validation and understanding felt. John Suchet (2010, p.198) recalls feelings of relief when being put in contact with a fellow carer, a retired headteacher of a similar age to him: '[It] makes such a nice change from all the people who say they know just how I feel because they have a relative with Alzheimer's, then it turns out they are in their eighties and nineties.'

This is a familiar sentiment in relation to those with young-onset dementia and it is concerning to note the lack of age-related services for those with young-onset dementia and their families.

Peer support interventions can improve carer well-being, and interventions that engage both the carer and person with dementia can have significant mutual benefits (Charlesworth *et al.* 2011). The BBC Two Wales documentary *Dementia: Making a Difference* (2012) was illustrative in regard to ways in which peer support groups can positively influence relationships between those with dementia and family members, providing welcome space for each party as well as new experiences to talk about. This reflects benefits noted elsewhere in this text of bringing family members together, having occasions to relate to each other more meaningfully and reinforcing relationships.

Dementia cafés

A notable example providing peer support for both those with dementia and family carers is a resource known as the dementia café or Alzheimer café. The first Alzheimer café was started by the Dutch psychiatrist Bere Miesen in the Netherlands in 1997 followed three years later by the opening of one in Farnborough, the first in the UK (Alzheimer Café Farnborough n.d.). An Alzheimer café involves monthly gatherings of people affected by dementia for the purposes of education, support, discussion, sharing experiences and exchanging information about dementia and local services as well as providing opportunities to socialize and meet others. The following list illustrates some of the discussion topics commonly addressed within Alzheimer cafés:

- behaviour changes and the variety of reasons for it (including fear, pain)
- explaining visuo-perceptual changes in dementia (and making environmental adaptations)
- how difficult is it to give up driving, and/or one's work?
- breaking through denial: what can help?
- how can receiving a diagnosis of dementia help you to 'move on'?
- how do you explain to others (neighbours, shopkeepers) that you have dementia?

The following daily ethical dilemmas have also been explored at some Alzheimer cafés:

- to lie or not to lie
- to help or let a person struggle a bit to do a thing or to help them quickly.

(www.alzheimercafe.co.uk)

It should be noted that there are various 'café models' in the UK currently operating, offered by different charities and groups. Whilst all meet social needs, the differing approaches include activities, generic talks, dementia education and support. They offer a safe, social setting to anyone and everyone interested in dementia, but particularly to people with dementia and their family and friends.

ACTIVITY 6.4

Do dementia café facilities exist within your locality, or not?

What could be the positives when attending such a café for:

- a person with dementia
- a carer/partner/friend
- the community.

Greenwood *et al.*'s (2017) thematic analysis identified four key elements relating to dementia cafés:

- Cafés provide a relaxed, welcoming atmosphere where carers feel supported and accepted.
- Café attendance often brought a sense of normality to these carers' lives.
- Carers and those they care for look forward to going and enjoy the activities provided and socializing with others.
- Other highlighted benefits included peer support from other carers, information provision and support from the volunteer café coordinators.

These aspects show some key functions for family dementia carers with the environment providing acceptance and welcome to those attending. Again, we hear of the support received from peers as well as the 'sense of normality' provided. This challenges stigmatizing attitudes and lowered expectations commonly associated with the dementia experience. We should not lose sight though of the fact that individuals with dementia and carers look forward to attending and gain enjoyment from activities engaged in. This will facilitate the coping with daily difficulties and provide a much-needed respite for all parties. The features identified here echo many of the findings in Capus's (2005) study, which suggested that dementia cafés provide an important venue for meeting others who are in a similar position, which helped to normalize the emotions that the experience of caring has evoked in them and the changes in relationships that have occurred since the onset of dementia. As Takechi *et al.* (2018) suggest, dementia cafés offer a strong type of community resource for dementia care in the present and future. This provides continuity of support and will help to anchor those concerned to something stable, especially with the changes taking place around and within their family groups.

A welcome sight is the appearance of dementia cafés geared towards supporting diversity. The Rainbow Café, the UK's first LGBT dementia café, provides those attending with non-judgemental assistance and a 'safe space to talk without having to explain their back stories' (Channel 4 2018). This concerns a societal group liable to experience discrimination and stigmatization on account of both their sexuality/sexual identity as well as their dementia. A participant of this dementia café remarked:

> There was an immediate sense of when we arrived in that group of people feeling that we were amongst friends…and trust which is a key need for many of us who are gay to feel that you can implicitly trust that others in the room are not going to judge you.

The expressed feeling of trust is crucial, especially relating to individuals and groups who are prone to feeling judged or negatively appraised. The further addition of a dementia diagnosis is liable to erode people's confidence and impact upon their sense of security when around others. Therefore, having an environment where individuals' sexuality need not become invisible, their dementia is accepted and understood and they can freely express themselves is clearly a very positive thing.

ACTIVITY 6.5

From your professional and/or personal experience, does discrimination and stigmatization happen when a person's sexuality/sexual identity are considered alongside their dementia?

Online peer support

A blossoming set of peer support resources can be found on the internet with key examples found within blogs, discussion forums and social media sites. These provide vibrant spaces for sharing and discussion around daily experience and topical themes. A noted feature within these resources concerns the duality of positions assumed by many participants engaged both in helping and supporting others as well as requesting help. These reciprocal roles reflect what might be regarded more as a position of 'normality' with a degree of agency or control resting with those getting involved.

BLOGS

A vibrant platform for experience sharing, as outlined in Gill's narrative, is that of blogging. The number of blogs written by carers and those with dementia continues to rise and the quality and expressive content contained in some of them is truly exceptional. These resources contextualize the dementia experience from a lived and felt perspective and put us very much in touch with ongoing daily occurrences, helping us appreciate something of what it *feels like* to experience dementia. It is as if we have a real-life soap opera being played out before us with characters we can strongly identify with and who are becoming increasingly familiar to us (Morris 2006). Such a degree of identification will promote connectedness and greater empathic understanding. Examples of high-quality bloggers in respect of persons with dementia include Kate Swaffer, Ken Clasper, Wendy Mitchell, Valerie Blumenthal, Chris Roberts, Silverfox and Howard Glick; and for carers we can review blogs by Linda Fischer, Sheri Zschocher, Kay Bransford, Jon Pollard and Bee (see Box 6.1 for examples).

BOX 6.1 BLOGS

PERSON WITH DEMENTIA

Kate Swaffer – Creating Life with Words (http://kateswaffer.com/2013/03/29/reactions-to-dementia)

Chris Roberts – Dementia Survivor So Far (https://mason4233.wordpress.com)

Howard Glick – FTD (fronto-temporal dementia) Dementia Support blog (http://earlydementiasupport.blogspot.co.uk)

Ken Clasper – Living Well with Lewy Body Disease (http://ken-kenc2.blogspot.co.uk)

Truthful Loving Kindness (http://truthfulkindness.com)

Silverfox – Sharing My Life with Lewy Body Dementia (http://parkblog-silverfox.blogspot.co.uk)

Wendy Mitchell – Which Me Am I Today (https://whichmeamitoday.wordpress.com/blog)

Valerie Blumenthal – Wise Words Lost Forever (https://wisewordslostforwords.wordpress.com)

Young Dementia UK (www.youngdementiauk.org/resources/blogs)

CARERS AND FAMILY MEMBERS

Linda Fischer – Early Onset Alzheimer's blog (http://earlyonset.blogspot.com)

Sheri Zschocher – Living in the Shadow of Alzheimer's…Goin' Through the Motions (http://sherizeee.blogspot.com)

Kay Bransford – Dealing with Dementia (https://dealingwithdementia.wordpress.com)

Jon Pollard – We Need Toothpaste (http://weneedtoothpaste.blogspot.com)

Bee – Her Absent Mind (http://herabsentmind.blogspot.com)

Kate Swaffer's blog 'Creating Life with Words: Inspiration, Love and Truth' is a wonderfully expressive resource with its author acting as a strong advocate for those living with dementia. Swaffer (2016, p.284) reflects upon the value in maintaining such a blog for herself and others, citing the many wonderful 'pen pals' afforded her and its potency in keeping depression at bay: 'Blogging and writing have opened up my world and my heart and definitely allowed me to be more discerning and to love myself more…also feel like positive psychosocial intervention, as well as non-pharmacological interventions for dementia.'

Her 'pen pals' are clearly more than mere correspondents, helping to foster and enhance feelings of self-worth. The statement 'allowed me…to love myself more' through non-pharmacological interventions strikes powerfully and offers much hope for people striving to live well with dementia. It shows how empowered individuals with dementia can become in pursuing and maintaining their own mood state and overall well-being. Another core feature of blogging noted by Swaffer (2016) includes the capacity to build up a memory bank of thoughts and to store accounts of life experiences and daily encounters. This is a fascinating notion, with a blog acting not only as a diary but also in a sense an external hard drive, capturing experience, discussion and moments of reflection from those sharing information and those responding to blog posts.

Blogging is described by Merchant (2004) as a valuable new way to share dementia knowledge. We can look at the Alzheimer's Society blog for examples with its platform for sharing stories and narratives from a number of people. A notable feature within these blogs concerns the opportunities for engagement between those posting and those responding to blogs. For example 'Sarah's Story', in connection with her father's dementia, was entitled 'I slowly realised I was losing my best friend' (Alzheimer's Society 2019b). Responses included:

- 'Beautiful words from a loving daughter.'
- 'Heartbreaking! What a lovely Dad you had!'
- 'Thank you so much for this Sarah, it moved me to tears. My sisters and I are going through this journey with our mother and your words have really helped.'

We can appreciate the comfort and sense of understanding that each party will feel in turn. Sarah is provided with an acknowledgement of her experience and validation of feelings from those reading her post. The respondents in turn are clearly evidencing something of how moved and connected they felt through Sarah's expression. This sense of engagement helps to tackle feelings of isolation and disconnectedness, but also helps individuals to validate their own feelings.

Dementia caregivers are also using blogs to share their experiences, posting rich narratives representing an untapped resource for understanding the psycho-social impact of caring for a person with dementia at the family level. A study by Anderson, Hundt and Dean (2016) examined blogs written by caregivers of persons with dementia. The four themes emerging from the narratives included information seeking, social support, reminiscing and altruism.

These themes reflect some of the benefits from blogging that relate to all family members. A fascinating feature within this study concerned the use of blogs as ways of updating family members and friends, with a caregiver noting: 'That was one reason I started this blog, so that friends and family could keep up with my mother's progression without me having to explain or discuss her disease.'

This is understandable given how hard (and distressing) it can be for those involved to share and explain the same information multiple times. Blogging also provides families with opportunities for all of its members to reach agreement on what they feel comfortable sharing with others.

Kannaley, Mehta and Yelta (2019) examined the types of information concerning the dementia experience being shared through blog posts. They selected 19 blogs written by people with Alzheimer's disease and related dementia and 44 blogs written by care partners. Thematic analysis of blog narratives generated a number of themes, including the impact that dementia has upon those concerned and personal experiences; identification of positive elements and coping mechanisms; feeling out of control; and issues connected with advocacy and empowerment.

These themes show the scope and range of personal experiences focusing upon both states of *struggling* and *coping*. Both caregivers and care recipients offered insight into their dementia experience and shared a variety of coping mechanisms. It is clear from the available evidence that blogs offer a valuable resource and promote a sense of community for those with dementia and their families. The range of groups represented by available blogs, though, could do with further development. Whilst there are blogs written for the LGBT or BME communities within advocacy groups such as the Alzheimer's Society and Alzheimer Scotland there is overall a paucity of available evidence.

DISCUSSION FORUMS

As with blogs, discussion forums provide opportunities for meaningful engagement with peers. Discussion forum members share stories, give advice and offer encouragement, as well as commiserating about their symptoms in ways that generate solidarity. It is a rich resource for narrative sharing that Rodriquez (2013) regards as essential not only for the construction of self, but also for the construction of community. This concept of community can be seen as vital for families prone to feeling progressively more isolated and disengaged from others. It is also important for the many people who for various reasons are finding it more difficult to leave their homes. There are a growing number of locations offering space for people to interact with like-minded people through online forums. Prominent examples include:

- Aging Care – www.agingcare.com/Alzheimers-Dementia/Discussions-1
- Alz Connected – www.alzconnected.org
- Alzheimer's Australia Discussion Forum – www.talkdementia.org.au

- Alzheimer's Society Talking Point Forum – http://forum.alzheimers.org.uk/forum.php
- Lewy Body Dementia Association – www.lbda.org/phpBB3/viewforum.php?f=10
- FTD Support Forum – www.ftdsupportforum.com.

A particular dynamic commonly noted with dementia discussion forums concerns the warm welcome offered to new members who are posting for the first time. For example, Arthur AsCII, who is new to the Alzheimer's Society's forum and announcing his diagnosis, is warmly responded to by fellow members. His subsequent reply is: 'Thank you. Seems like there are many, many good people around here' (Alzheimer's Society 2019c).

This signifies and acknowledges the safety and support available within this resource. Another post from Aitchkbee titled 'My Mum' expresses: 'Hello. I am really concerned about my mum. She is 72 and over the last few months her behaviour has changed considerably. She doesn't appear to have issues with her memory but can suddenly become aggressive and so angry' (Alzheimer's Society 2018b). Replies to this include advice and related experiences from others. This post stimulated a lively discussion amongst respondents and the person posting.

McKechnie, Barker and Stott's (2014) mixed methods study examined the impact of online support forum for carers of people with dementia. They found an improvement in the quality of the relationship with the person with dementia. Clearly, the reinforcement and nurturing of this relationship highlights the core value of this resource and is something that healthcare professionals need to be mindful of.

SOCIAL MEDIA

The final look at online resources within this section is concerned with the variety of resources that are considered as social media. As this term implies, they are concerned with information sharing, discussion and engagement amongst their members. As Craig and Strivens (2016) assert, Facebook provides a means of rapid global reach in a way that allows people with dementia to increase their communications and potentially reduce isolation. Such sites include a variety of advocacy groups with dementia organizations strongly featured. Box 6.2 provides examples of some of the main dementia groups that have created a shared space within various social media platforms.

BOX 6.2 FACEBOOK AND TWITTER

Children of Parents with Dementia

Dementia Family Connection

Forget Me Not Dementia Support Group

Alzheimer's Society

Dementia Friends

Dementia and Alzheimer UK Carers Group

Dementia Family Support

Alzheimer's Support Group for Family Friends

Dementia UK

Dementia Centre (Australia)

Alzheimer's and Dementia Support

Dementia Support

Lewy Body Dementia Carers

Alzheimer's Awareness

Dementia Awareness

Vascular Dementia UK

Young Dementia UK

Dementia Aware

A quick glance at Facebook and Twitter show the wide variety and range of dementia-related groups and organizations. For example, the Young Onset Dementia Support Group feature, on both platforms and provide followers with space to post comments, read educational information and related news feeds, share inspirational quotes and access others living with dementia worldwide. Robillard *et al.* (2013) examined the use of Twitter for sharing information about dementia. They reviewed over 9200 tweets, finding that a majority of them contained links to third-party sites rather than personal information. There were also a large number of tweets discussing recent research findings related to the prediction and risk management of Alzheimer's disease. Whilst providing a rich resource for information sharing, other social media platforms such as Facebook perhaps engage participants on a more personal level. A glance at the Alzheimer's Society's Facebook page shows a rich level of discussion, provision of support and sharing of experience.

The chosen channel for narrative sharing can be important for members where the written word is becoming more difficult to fathom. Dementia Diaries is a UK-wide project that brings together people's diverse experiences of living with dementia through audio diaries. It serves as a public record and a personal archive that documents the views, reflections and day-to-day lives of people living with dementia, with the aim of prompting dialogue and changing attitudes. The value of this online resource is outlined in the following narrative:

> I'm ever so grateful for Dementia Diaries where we are on Twitter and we're on Facebook and we all have buddies where we can support each other and ask any kind of question and it's not outlandish or anything and we feel safe. (Dementia Diaries 2018)

The examples of peer support available to individuals with dementia and their families illustrate a vibrant and vital set of resources. These provide opportunities for people to feel properly acknowledged and understood. A notable feature is the observation of those concerned operating through very different modes of engagement (illustrating both states of vulnerability and resilience), asking for help and support as well as providing this to others. The opportunity to help others will help to preserve individuals' feelings of value and personal importance, a powerful counter to the growing sense of helplessness and impotence commonly experienced. A notable feature connected with peer support resources is the level of autonomy and agency taken up by those with first-hand experience. This shows all too clearly Swaffer's (2016) notion of *living beyond dementia* and features prominently in the following section, which is concerned with creative and artistic modalities.

Creative arts (self-expression and therapeutic benefits) ('Finding my voice')

There is a real need to consider the richness and vitality of communicative forms that offer additional means of conveying concepts, feelings and experiences. This is especially important given the restrictions many people will be experiencing in relation to their expression of words. The many benefits offered from creative modalities to those with dementia include the means of promoting self, a reawakening of personal identity and a vehicle for stimulation and feeling truly alive. The creative arts cover a wide variety of types including art, music, poetry and dance. They offer immense value not only to those with dementia but also partners and wider family members. Lepp *et al.* (2003) reports upon a cultural drama programme focusing on dance, rhythm, song, storytelling and conversations for patients with dementia and their caregivers. The categories, 'interaction' and 'professional growth', emerged from the analysis with caregivers describing the development of fellowship with other participants and the sharing of both joy and sorrow. The patients also connected meaningfully with others, were stimulated to recall memories and demonstrated aspects of themselves unknown by carers.

From a practice point of view such approaches tend to be overlooked with many opportunities to facilitate communication and self-expression missed. Aadlandsvik (2000) disputes Plato's hierarchy of knowledge, which considers mathematical thought to be the highest and the arts the most basic. Indeed, there are current concerns over the decline of arts-based subjects within the National Curriculum with a decreasing number of pupils studying art, drama or music (*The Guardian* 2018). It is not surprising therefore to find a similar picture within healthcare with art therapies and creative modalities relegated somewhere far behind medical interventions. A potential occurrence within residential homes and in-patient settings might be locked cupboards with art equipment and materials gathering dust. What entertainment or creative approaches there are may be carelessly selected with, for example, musical entertainers of variable quality playing (perhaps badly) to *captive* audiences. The issue here concerns *choice* and the degree to which personal preferences are consulted or attended to. Creative approaches need to be carefully considered and targeted directly towards the unique interests and passions of each individual.

Gill's Narrative 6.3: The arts are amazing

'The art group we go to is simply fabulous and it is great to see Peter so animated and at peace with himself. We have regular outings to art galleries as well as attending still-life classes. They are a nice group of people, mostly couples, and it is refreshing to spend time socializing. What is most amazing is an expression I often hear – "You can't really tell who has dementia." I would echo that as when Peter is painting or drawing he seems to be engrossed and relaxed with his usual agitation or restlessness seemingly gone.

I feel very close to Peter during these activities and we both look forward to the group meetings very much. This is something we share and that brings us together, reaffirming our relationship as husband and wife.'

■ *What benefits do you think Gill is getting from these group activities?*

■ *What benefits could Peter be experiencing from these group activities?*

Gill's narrative shows the renewed animation and heightened well-being that can be promoted through creative activities. As illustrated, the benefits are not only felt by those with dementia but also family members with experiences and events that can be eagerly looked forward to and that help to strengthen familial relationships. Gill also notes Peter's reduced agitation and restlessness whilst engaged in activities, something that McGreevy's (2016) review found with arts-based and creative approaches to dementia care recognized as a viable alternative to antipsychotic medication. As well as highlighting the success of these activities they also outlined the lack of negative side-effects.

Arts-based interventions have a rich expressive function providing valuable and broad channels of communication. In relation to people with dementia, the writer and poet John Killick noted that whilst language was not always easy to interpret in conventional terms, it had a metaphorical richness and used images that could, with the right kind of encouragement and attention, convey powerful messages (Killick and Allan 2001). As Kitwood and Bredin (1992, p.27) asserted:

> We may need to develop special skills in order to understand what a confused person is trying to get across...the best thing is to treat everything they say, however jumbled or fantastic it may seem to be, as an attempt to tell us something. Look for the message that underlies the words, or a need that is being expressed. Get a sense of the feeling that is coming across with the words.

The *special skills* and interventions indicated here are already being used within dementia care through some inspirational projects and initiatives. These provide modes for individuals to communicate with others and to express what is central to their experience. This will be examined within this section in relation to:

- art
- music and singing
- poetry and creative writing
- dance.

Art

Whilst the term 'art' can be regarded as applying to an extensive sensory range, the focus in this instance is mainly upon the visual concept, which includes painting, drawing and sculpture. For people with dementia experiencing cognitive and communicative deficits, art provides a valuable means of self-expression and engagement with others. When offered as art therapy it can be regarded as:

> A process which allows individuals, in a space in which they cannot be wrong or make mistakes, to explore through images their hopes and fears and memories. The images may be painted, drawn, made as a collage or by using words. (Baines 2011, p.124)

The 'space in which they cannot be wrong or make mistakes' is of vital importance, especially given the increasingly regular experience of struggling to find and convey the right words, observing the bemused confusion on the faces of others or enduring the frustration and humiliation of being frequently corrected. Through art there is real freedom to express self as well as having one's vital communication accepted and validated by others. Opportunities to participate in artistic and creative expression in group settings can be beneficial to health and well-being (Hannemann 2006) and we can also acknowledge improvements in mood with art therapy helping to alleviate feelings of depression (Rusted, Sheppard and Waller 2006). Indeed, the potency of art as an expressive medium for those with dementia can be regarded as transformative as shown by John Zeisel (2008):

> It is quite amazing how art can help. It actually reduces the symptoms of the illness, and it reduces some of the behaviours that people associate with Alzheimer's that aren't really direct symptoms but people see as symptoms… When people are engaged with art, whether it is visual art at the museum or circus art or poetry, they can focus attention for much, much longer.

This covers some essential points including the significantly increased level of attention and focus that can be applied to activities. This extended attention will also facilitate productivity and subsequently help foster satisfaction, enjoyment, engagement and well-being.

The text *I Remember Better When I Paint* (Huebner 2012) illustrates how art can reach areas of emotion, creativity and expression and reflects the powerful transformation that can be experienced. The Art Gallery Access Programme investigated the effect of taking people with dementia to discuss artworks at the National Gallery of Australia. During these visits, participants became animated, gained confidence and were able to discuss and interact with the artworks and the social process. This included the more impaired groups, who were more withdrawn or behaviourally disturbed elsewhere in their usual environment (MacPherson *et al.* 2009). Another related project is Meet Me at MoMA. The Museum of Modern Art and the New York University Center of Excellence for Brain Aging and Dementia completed an evaluative study of their arts innovation. Their findings demonstrated engagement with arts programmes improving mood for both people with dementia and family carers (Rosenberg *et al.* 2009).

Music and singing

Robertson-Gillam (2011, p.96) promotes the potency of singing within dementia care: 'We all have a voice and this can be transformed into a creative communicative device when ordinary speech fails.' What this statement alludes to is the recognition of the *voice* that people with dementia retain along with the provision of a means for that voice to be 'heard'. This challenges the common perception of communicative disability in relation to individuals' restrictive use of words. Music can also be seen to have a powerfully therapeutic calming effect. The Alzheimer's Society (2019a) report upon the carpool karaoke Songaminute Man (Ted McDermott, former Butlin's Redcoat with dementia) and the video of him that went viral. His son Simon commented upon the increase in aggressive behaviour caused by Ted's deteriorating cognitive state. Singing provided welcome moments of relief for the family where it was noticed: 'He's a lot happier – it takes him back to his passion. There are still dark days, but it's better than it was... After singing his conversation is much better. He'll talk about his music.'

Clift *et al.* (2008) found some evidence in their review that group singing had a positive effect on mood in relation to:

- emotional release and reduction of feelings of stress
- a sense of happiness, positive mood, joy, elation and feeling high
- a sense of greater personal, emotional and physical well-being
- increased self-confidence and self-esteem.

We might also here reflect upon the group singing projects in Vicky McClure's documentary *Our Dementia Choir* (2019) or Gareth Malone's *The Choir* with participants routinely expressing enhancements to their self-confidence and mood states.

ACTIVITY 6.6

Think of a song that has fond memories for you.

- What is the song and when did you first hear it?
- When you now hear this song, what memories and feelings does it conjure up?

Further evidence of positive impact is provided by Clarkson, Cassidy and Eskes (2007) through their examination of non-pharmacological strategies for managing the behavioural and psychological symptoms of dementia. Music programmes were found to impact positively upon levels of agitation and stimulated communication amongst residents. This illustrates the soothing capacity of music and singing.

Music can also act as a memory aid helping to preserve personal identity. As Jenkins (2014) asserts, music acts as a mnemonic device that can evoke experiences and emotions. Indeed, the use of music for connecting memories to times in a person's life or emotions associated with memories provides an important vehicle for promoting personhood. The charitable organisation Playlist for Life invites people to 'find the soundtrack to your life' by compiling a unique collection of songs that have a personal resonance to a time, place or a person. For carers, music can provide an important therapeutic bridge to their emotional experience. Robertson-Gillam (2011) provides an arresting example of a carer within counselling identifying a song that enabled her to reframe and understand the complex feelings she held towards her husband.

McDermott, Orrell and Ridder's study (2014) identified a core strength through music engagement with closer links being forged between personal identity and life events. This was recognized through their theme 'Who you are now':

> Music gives him a kind of wholeness, of a person, of his spirituality, life generally. Probably connects him with some of his earlier life in a way of how he saw life. Music takes him back to the times he was able to be himself.

The potency of music is further illustrated by participants in their study:

> I think music always brings back their memory. Remembering old songs… you can see changes [in residents]. Resident E starts dancing…once he told me 'that's not the way you dance' so he started teaching me how to dance. (Susan, staff member)

> Resident A whistles…legs going, waving her hands…her knowledge of music is incredible, because she can whistle anything, even though her memory is poor, she can even whistle the Blaydon races that I hadn't played [on CD]…she remembers. (Stephen, staff member)
>
> [I] forget things…but when I make a cup of tea standing in the kitchen, I sing what I remember. Music when I was a child, I am old now, but music [stays]. (Peter, day hospital client) (McDermott, Orrell, and Ridder 2014)

These narratives shows something of the reaffirmation a person can achieve regarding their 'earlier life'. It starkly illustrates how detached a person with dementia can feel and how important such a spiritual reawakening of self can be. Indeed, Austin (1999) regards music as creating links to an individual's core being and serving to connect people to breath, physicality and emotion. A striking example of this can be seen in the film *Alive Inside* showing 92-year-old Henry Dryer's sudden animation when played music by artists dear to him such as Cab Calloway or Bing Crosby. The noted neurologist Oliver Sacks, author of *Awakenings*, reflected: 'We first see Henry inert, maybe depressed, unresponsive and almost unalive…then he is given an iPod containing his favourite music… And immediately he lights up' (Moisse 2012).

What seems to be miraculous really serves to alert us to the evident need to reach out to those with dementia, no matter how severely they appear to be affected. This allows opportunities for them to bridge the gap between worlds that might be becoming increasingly closed and inaccessible. Here we have a person in what we might regard as the severe or late-stage of their dementia, seemingly disengaged and uncommunicative, moved albeit momentarily to a state of animation, expressiveness and energy. The joy of this transformation is clearly seen on the faces of his family members with their loved one restored to them.

Another core feature with music is the opportunity to feel connected and engaged with the person with dementia. As illustrated in Robertson-Gillam's (2011) case study:

> Betsy was in the late stages of dementia and had lost the ability to communicate verbally. She regularly wandered up and down the corridor of the nursing home vocalising like an opera singer loudly and constantly. I joined her one day and matched the pace of her steps. As our rhythm became synchronised Betsy looked at me and smiled… We walked the length of the nursing home together singing back and forth. Betsy became more reflective and attentive, nodding and saying 'yes, yes' … Betsy just needed someone to recognise her innate self and she was satisfied.

This narrative illustrates a profound sense of connection between two people who for an instant are properly in tune with each other. Betty's subsequent feelings of contentedness are evidently stimulated through the sense of recognition and validation attained here.

The benefits of music can be extended to couples' (person with dementia and family carer) relationships as evidenced by Unadkat, Camic and Vella-Burrows' (2017) study. They interviewed 17 couples, finding group singing experienced as joyful and promoting active participation. The benefits were experienced for each person individually as well as for them as a couple through participation in new experiences and enhancements in their relationship.

It is pleasing to note the growing number of emerging projects such as Lost Chord, set up by a Yorkshire-based charity and aiming to enhance the social and emotional well-being of people with dementia through interaction with musical stimuli. Likewise, the Music for Thought project is an interactive, therapeutic music workshop programme with professional musicians and students playing alongside people affected by dementia.

Poetry and creative writing

There are some very inspiring literary projects helping to provide those with dementia with a means of expression and engagement with their external world. A particular example, Mind's Eye Poetry, was founded by Molly Meyer in 2013 in Dallas, Texas. The aims of this project are to help those with dementia access memories and imagination by utilizing ideas, phrases, words and even non-verbal cues. 'To hear someone speak who hasn't said a word in weeks, or to watch tears of joy rush down someone's face because they've remembered something long forgotten is the greatest feeling in the world' (Alzheimer's Net 2017).

ACTIVITY 6.7

Do you have a favourite book or poem?

Why does this writing retain a meaningful place in your memories?

For those in advanced stages, Meyer brings sensory props to look at, touch and listen to, which relate to the poems she's reciting, and provides another dimension of cognitive stimulation. She comments upon the striking sense of *awakening* which occurs with previously uncommunicative patients subsequently expressing themselves with real vitality and meaning.

The key word here is *awakening*, showing the person's re-engagement with their external world, communicating with meaning and gaining validation from others. This is a welcome change for many people from the increasing restrictiveness and solitude of their internal sphere.

Aadlandsvik (2000) reports upon a project exploring the impact of creative writing and storytelling for people with early dementia. The findings demonstrated enhanced communication and engagement between participants. The themes expressed showed depth of maturity covering loss and suffering, delight, dance and joy, friendship and loneliness, good and evil, as well as the 'mystery of life'. This project utilized an innovative approach involving co-creation, which also formed the basis of the Alzheimer's Poetry Project (Swinnen 2016). It positioned people with dementia as co-creators of embodied texts, which were subsequently read by a poet-performer, validating the words that the participants contributed. It is in the ongoing exchange between performer and audience who simultaneously produce and consume poetry that comfort is found, not only for the people with dementia but for the poet-performer as well.

Clark-McGhee and Castro (2015) conducted a narrative analysis of meaning-making within poems from the words of people diagnosed with dementia. Narratives powerfully highlighted the depth of expressiveness with some striking elements communicated. It evidenced individuals' lack of agency over their experiences connected with received care. It also highlighted a repositioning and reframing by others of a person's identity constructs. Lastly, it showed the importance of acknowledging and supporting 'personhood' in order to strengthen well-being and individuals' sense of purpose.

The first point gives health carers much food for thought with *lack of agency* being created more through care approaches than the person's dementia. We also see new identity constructs being created for those with dementia that can be at odds with who the person essentially is. Lastly, the value of personhood is affirmed. These are all vital elements and show the need to facilitate communication and attend more vigorously to what people with dementia are expressing.

Dance

Rambert, Britain's oldest dance company, offer specialized dance sessions for people in the early stages of dementia. Their workshops comprise of warm-ups, partner and group exercises, dance and a chance to explore steps from Rambert's repertoire to stimulate movement memory. Amongst the positive feedback for these classes, the following statement shows the impact upon well-being: 'It would be useful to have these on a year round basis. They have a noticeable improvement in the general well-being of my husband, especially in his mood and engagement with music' (Rambert n.d.).

Elements that stand out here are the noted improvements in both *well-being* and *mood.* Also, the *year round basis* comment does show the value in maintenance of approaches that have a discernible and positive impact upon participants. There are related initiatives being offered by Edinburgh's Dance Base in Scotland and Caernarfon's *Dawns i Bawb* (Dance for All) in Wales with the health benefits outlined in the All-Party Parliamentary Group on Arts, Health and Wellbeing Inquiry (2017). This report illustrates how engagement with the arts including dancing can boost brain function, stimulate recall of memories and improve the quality of life for people with dementia and their families.

The findings of a two-year research study exploring the impact on quality of life and well-being of the dance movement programme Remember to Dance (2013) for people in different stages of dementia included the observations:

- enjoyment
- maintained levels of involvement
- improved vitality
- progressively freer and more fluid physical movements
- creative expression relating to types of activities
- manifestations of self in the here and now
- positive social interactions and social bonding
- positive relationships between carers and their cared-for
- improved or supported well-being/positive mood
- nurtured issues of choice and confidence
- states of prolonged satisfaction/achievement/confidence
- reduction of listlessness/distress.

(Vella-Burrows and Wilson 2016)

Some participants of this programme were observed to become more animated and engaged as various props were added towards the end of the session. There were also reported benefits from the social element with new friendships established (reported by a Remember to Dance in the Community dancer).

Hayes (2011) reports upon the benefits experienced through a movement session involving touch, enabling individuals to reach out and feel connected with others: 'As we feel cut off because of the disjointed world we begin to withdraw into our own bodies. Reaching out less and less.'

What this narrative stresses is the crucial need to feel in touch (across all holistic domains) with other people. For many people with dementia this can start to feel more elusive, progressively retreating further inwardly. Meaningful connection with others is spiritually nurturing, validates our sense of existence in the world and helps us to feel alive.

This section highlighted a number of issues with regard to dementia care and the potency of employing creative and innovative approaches. As has been noted though repeated narrative observations, there can be a sense of 're-awakening' for those with dementia who are brought back into the 'here and now' through their exposure to creative and artistic stimuli. The benefits here can be felt by many individuals with carers and family members feeling reconnected with loved ones and sharing important moments of intimacy together. In essence, it shows us that there are many opportunities for employing methods and approaches that resonate meaningfully with those we are working with and enable the 'humanness' of individuals with dementia, no matter their level of cognitive deterioration, to be acknowledged and nurtured.

How true could this be today?

The theme of 'How true could this be today?' asks you to consider reframing an observation from the past. This commentary had an influence in informing thinking at that time whilst also determining opinions of the day. A number of questions will encourage you to consider its relevance in the here and now, such as: have national opinions changed or not? Do you agree or not with these comments? What has influenced your attitudes?

Background information: the work of Tom Kitwood and the Bradford Dementia Group during the concluding decades of the twentieth century were challenging the 'older order' of dementia care with its reliance on traditional institutionalized approaches. They advocated a more humanistic and person-centred philosophy.

The final 'How true could this be today?' is based upon ways of thinking about uniqueness. Kitwood (1997) asked for dementia to be reconsidered and posited that a person's uniqueness can be regarded through a number of dimensions including their culture, gender, temperament, social class, lifestyle, outlook, beliefs, values, commitments, tastes and interests.

- Some two decades on, do you feel his views promote a better understanding of a person's uniqueness?
- What has previously influenced your attitudes to dementia and its care?
- Have you found that your views have changed over time or not?
- Based upon your above responses, what types of mutual interventions could encourage this uniqueness?

Concluding thoughts

This chapter acts as a balance and counter to the related difficulties and 'struggles' outlined within previous chapters. The core themes powerfully remind us that people continue to exist and have something vital to offer to others despite a steady advancement of their symptoms. Swaffer's (2016) concept of *living beyond dementia* is a potent reminder of people's continued lives and roles and the fact that they need not become totally defined by their diagnosis. With the right level and type of support, people with dementia and their families can continue to assert their individual and collective identities. Peer support offers immense value through helping people to feel heard, acknowledged, comforted and connected with those who truly understand. It also enables those involved to offer their own solace and support, thereby reaffirming and validating what they themselves can give of worth. Finally, the creative arts provide further opportunities for those concerned to deal proactively with stress, promote well-being and discover modes that facilitate communication. The interventions and approaches covered in this chapter are deliberately chosen and relate very much to what individuals, families and dementia advocacy groups are themselves involved in or running. There is a real sense here of autonomy and hope, led by those who know best what it feels like to live with dementia. The positivity attained here continues into the next chapter, which acknowledges people, campaigns, resources, initiatives, environmental modifications and societal responses that can rightly be regarded as 'dementia champions'.

PERSONAL LEARNING

What was your past knowledge and understanding, what new learning have you achieved and how could this inform your future personal and/or professional interventions?

As a 'family member', my new learning includes ....

....

On reading the first-person narratives, my new learning includes

....

INTERVENTIONS

Be mindful that whatever comments are offered should be realistic, achievable and person-centred. Also, that the feelings conveyed and observations made reinforce the 'coping approaches experienced' for the individual and significant other people in their life.

The types of intervention could include ....

....

References

Aadlandsvik, R. (2000). 'The second sight: learning about and with dementia by means of poetry.' *The International Journal of Social Research* 7 (3), 321–329.

Aging Care (n.d.). *Alzheimer's and Dementia Care.* Accessed on 18/3/19 at www.agingcare.com/Alzheimers-Dementia/Discussions-1.

All-Party Parliamentary Group on Arts, Health and Wellbeing Inquiry (2017). *Creative Health: The Arts for Health and Wellbeing.* Accessed on 2/6/18 at www.artshealthandwellbeing.org.uk/appg-inquiry/Publications/Creative_Health_The_Short_Report.pdf.

Alz Connected (n.d.). *Alz Connected.* Accessed on 18/3/19 at www.alzconnected.org.

Alzheimer Café Farnborough (n.d.). *Alzheimer Café Farnborough: All in the Same Boat.* Accessed on 9/1/20 at www.alzheimercafe.co.uk/Farnborough.htm.

Alzheimer's Disease International (2016). *Dementia Friendly Communities: Key Principles.* Accessed on 7/9/17 at www. alz.co.uk/adi/pdf/dfc-principles.

Alzheimer's Net (2017). *Mind's Eye Poetry.* Accessed on 15/4/18 at www.alzheimers.net/3-25-15-minds-eye-poetry-for-dementia.

Alzheimer's Society (2018a). *We are the storm: the power of a shared voice.* Accessed on 6/7/19 at www.alzheimers.org.uk/dementia-together-magazine/dec-jan-2018-2019/we-are-storm-power-shared-voice.

Alzheimer's Society (2018b). *My Mum.* Accessed on 27/10/19 at https://forum.alzheimers.org.uk/threads/my-mum.113394/#post-1597335.

Alzheimer's Society (2019a). *Pride of Britain: The Story Behind the Songaminute Man Sensation*. Accessed on 13/12/19 at www.alzheimers.org.uk/get-support/publications-and-factsheets/dementia-together-magazine/pride-britain-story-behind.

Alzheimer's Society (2019b). *Sarah's Story: I Slowly Realised I was Losing My Best Friend*. Accessed on 22/3/19 at www.alzheimers.org.uk/blog/sarahs-story-i-slowly-realised-i-was-losing-my-best-friend.

Alzheimer's Society (2019c). *Alzheimer's it it then...* Accessed on 27/10/19 at https://forum.alzheimers.org.uk/threads/alzheimers-it-it-then.113820.

Anderson, J., Hundt, E. and Dean, M. (2016). 'The Church of Online Support: examining the use of blogs among family caregivers of persons with dementia.' *Journal of Family Nursing 23* (1), 34–54.

Austin, D. (1999). 'Vocal improvisation in analytically oriented music therapy with adults.' In T. Wigram and J. De Backer (eds) *Clinical Applications of Music Therapy in Psychiatry*. London: Jessica Kingsley Publishers.

Baines, P. (2011). 'Art Therapy and Dementia Care.' In H. Lee and T. Adams (eds) *Creative Approaches in Dementia Care*. London: Palgrave MacMillan.

BBC (2019). 'Why should I stop working just because I have dementia?' 27 September. Accessed on 19/11/19 at www.bbc.co.uk/news/stories-49745526.

BBC One (1993). *Link*. 8 October.

BBC One (2019). *Our Dementia Choir with Vicky McClure*. 2 May.

BBC Radio 4 (2019). *Woman's Hour*. 2 April.

BBC Two Wales (2012). *Dementia: Making a Difference*. 24 May.

Bryden, C. (2005). *Dancing with Dementia*. London: Jessica Kingsley Publishers.

Bryden, C. (2015). *Nothing About Us, Without Us! 20 Years of Dementia Advocacy*. London: Jessica Kingsley Publishers.

Bryden, C. (2018). *Will I Still Be Me? Finding a Continuing Sense of Self in the Lived Experience of Dementia*. London: Jessica Kingsley Publishers.

Capus, J. (2005). 'The Kingston Dementia Café: the benefits of establishing an Alzheimer café for carers and people with dementia.' *The International Journal of Social Research and Practice 4* (4), 588–591.

Channel 4 (2018). *Rainbow Café*. 21 April.

Channel 4 (2019). *The Restaurant That Makes Mistakes*. 12 June.

Charlesworth, G., Burnell, K., Beecham, J., Hoare, Z., Hoe, J., Wenborn, J., Knapp, M., Russell, I., Woods, B. and Orrell, M. (2011). 'Peer support for family carers of people with dementia, alone or in combination with group reminiscence in a factorial design: study protocol for a randomised controlled trial.' *Trials 12*, 205.

Clare, L., Nelis, S., Quinn, C., Martyr, A., Henderson, C., Hindle, J., Jones, I., Jones. R., Knapp, M., Kopelman, M., Morris, R., Pickett, J., Rusted, J., Savitch, N., Thom, J. and Victor, C. (2014). 'Improving the experience of dementia and enhancing active life – living well with dementia: study protocol for the IDEAL study.' *Health and Quality of Life Outcomes 12* (164), 1–15.

Clark-McGhee, K. and Castro, M. (2015). 'A narrative analysis of poetry written from the words of people given a diagnosis of dementia.' *Dementia 14* (1), 9–26.

Clarkson, K., Cassidy, K. and Eskes, G. (2007). 'Singing soothes: music concerts for the management of agitation in older adults with dementia.' *Canadian Journal of Geriatrics 10* (3), 80–87.

Clift, S., Hancox, G., Staricoff, R. and Whitmore, C. (2008). *Singing and Health: A Systematic Mapping and Review of Non-Clinical Research*. Canterbury: Sidney De Haan Research Centre for Arts and Health.

Craig, D. and Strivens, E. (2016). 'Facing the times: a young onset dementia support group: Facebook style.' *Australasian Journal on Ageing 35* (1), 48–53.

Dementia Diaries (2018). *Jacqui values the peer support she gets from social media and dementia diaries. She also wishes that support for others*. Accessed on 25/10/19 at www.dementiadiaries.org/entry/9760/jacui-values-the-peer-support-she-gets-from-social-media-and-dementia-diaries-she-also-wishes-that-support-for-others.

Dementia Together (2019). *Bang the Drum*. Accessed on 23/10/19 at www.alzheimers.org.uk/sites/default/files/2019-05/Dementiatogether_JuneJuly2019.pdf.

Department of Health and Social Care (2009). *Living Well with Dementia: A National Dementia Strategy*. London: Department of Health and Social Care.

FTD Support Forum (n.d.). *FTD Support Forum*. Accessed on 3/9/18 at www.ftdsupportforum.com.

Genova, L. (2007). *Still Alice*. New York: Simon and Schuster.

Greenwood, N., Smith, R., Akhtar, F. and Richardson, A. (2017). 'A qualitative study of carers' experiences of dementia cafés: a place to feel supported and be yourself.' *BMC Geriatrics 17* (1), 164.

Guardian, The (2018). 'Secret Teacher: subjects like art are being sidelined – but they matter.' 6 January. Accessed on 22/8/19 at www.theguardian.com/teacher-network/2018/jan/06/secret-teacher-unbalanced-curriculum-sats-assessment-children-art-music-languages-sidelined.

Hannemann, B. (2006). 'Creativity with dementia patients: can creativity and art stimulate dementia patients positively?' *Gerontology 52*, 59–65.

Hayes, J. (2011). *The Creative Arts in Dementia Care*. London: Jessica Kingsley Publishers.

Health Innovation Network (2015). *Peer Support for People with Dementia Resource Pack*. London: Health Innovation Network.

Huebner, B. (ed.). (2012). *I Remember Better When I Paint*. Echo Falls: Bethesda Communication Group.

Ignatieff, M. (1993). *Scar Tissue*. New York: Farrar, Straus and Giroux.

Jenkins, T. (2014). *Why does music evoke memories?* Accessed on 4/7/19 at www.bbc.com/culture/story/20140417-why-does-music-evoke-memories.

Kannaley, K., Mehta, S. and Yelta, B. (2019). 'Thematic analysis of blog narratives written by people with Alzheimer's disease and other dementias and care partners.' *Dementia 18* (7–8), 3071–3090.

Keyes, S., Clarke, C., Wilkinson, H., Alexjuk, E., Wilcockson, J., Robinson, L., Reynolds, J., McClelland, S., Corner, L. and Cattan, M. (2016). '"We're all thrown in the same boat." A qualitative analysis of peer support in dementia care.' *Dementia 15* (4), 560–577.

Killick, J. and Allan, K. (2001). *Communication and the Care of People with Dementia*. Buckingham: Open University Press.

Kitwood, T. (1997). *Dementia Reconsidered*. Maidenhead: Open University Press.

Kitwood, T, and Bredin, K. (1992). *Person to Person: Guide to the Care of Those with Failing Mental Powers*. London: Gale Centre Publications.

Kozberg, C. (n.d). *A Jewish Response to Dementia: Honoring Broken Tablets*. Accessed on 3/12/19 at www.caregiverslibrary.org/portals/0/Microsoft%20Word%20-%20A%20Jewish%20Response%20to%20Dementia[1].pdf.

Lauritzen, J., Pedersen, P.U., Sorensen, E.E. and Bjerrum, M.B. (2015). 'The meaningfulness of participating in support groups for informal caregivers of older adults with dementia: a systematic review.' *JBI Database of Systematic Reviews and Implementation Reports 13* (6), 373–433.

Lepp, M., Ringsberg, K., Holm, A. and Sellersjö, G. (2003). 'Dementia – involving patients and their caregivers in a drama programme: the caregivers' experiences.' *Journal of Clinical Nursing 12* (6), 873–881.

Lewy Body Dementia Association (n.d.). *Lewy Body Dementia Association*. Accessed on 16/6/18 at www.lbda.org/phpbbforum.

Lost Chord (n.d.). *Lost Chord*. Accessed on 12/2/18 at https://lost-chord.co.uk.

MacPherson, S., Bird, M., Anderson, K., Davis, T. and Blair, A. (2009). 'An art gallery access programme for people with dementia: "you do it for the moment".' *Aging Mental Health 13* (5), 744–752.

McDermott, O., Orrell, M. and Ridder, H. (2014). 'The importance of music for people with dementia: the perspectives of people with dementia, family carers, staff and music therapists.' *Aging and Mental Health 18* (6), 706–716.

McGreevy, J. (2016). 'Arts-based and creative approaches to dementia care.' *Nursing Older People 28* (1), 20–23.

McKechnie, V., Barker, C. and Stott, J. (2014). 'The effectiveness of an internet support forum for carers of people with dementia: a pre-post cohort study.' *Journal of Medical Internet Research 16* (2), e68.

Merchant, R. (2004). 'Go Forth and Blog.' *Journal of Dementia Care 12* (5), 12.

Moisse, K. (2012). *Alzheimer's Disease: Music Brings Patients 'Back to Life.'* Accessed on 10/5/19 at www.abcnews.go.com/Health/AlzheimersCommunity/alzheimers-disease-music-brings-patients-back-life/story?id=16117602.

Moriarty, J., Sharif, N. and Robinson, J. (2011). *SCIE Research Briefing 35: Black and Minority Ethnic People with Dementia and Their Access to Support and Services*. London: Social Care Institute for Excellence.

Mitchell, W. (2018). *Somebody I Used to Know*. London: Bloomsbury.

Morris, G. (2006). *Mental Health Issues and the Media*. London: Routledge.

Morris, G. (2017). *The Lived Experience in Mental Health*. London: CRC Press.

Music for Thought (n.d.). *Music for Thought*. Accessed on 13/2/17 at https://wigmore-hall.co.uk.

Newman, R. and Price, E. (2012). 'Meeting the Needs of LGBT People Affected by Dementia: The Story LGBT Dementia Support Group.' In R. Ward, I. Rivers and M. Sutherland (eds) *Lesbian, Gay, Bisexual and Transgender Ageing*. London: Jessica Kingsley Publishers.

Playlist for Life (n.d.). *Playlist for Life*. Accessed on 15/5/17 at https://playlistforlife.org.uk.

Rabanal, L., Chatwin, J., Walker, A., O'Sullivan, M. and Williamson, T. (2018). 'Understanding the needs and experiences of people with young onset dementia: a qualitative study.' *BMJ Open 8*: e021166.

Rambert (n.d.). *My wonderful experience as Elder's Programme Co-ordinator*. Accessed on 16/9/19 at www.rambert.org.uk.

Remember to Dance (2013). *Remember to Dance!* Accessed on 27/6/18 at www.greencandledance.com/2013/11/27/remember-to-dance.

Robertson-Gillam, K. (2011). 'Music Therapy in Dementia Care.' In H. Lee and T. Adams (eds) *Creative Approaches in Dementia Care*. London: Palgrave MacMillan.

Robillard, J., Johnson, T., Hennessey, C., Beattie, B. and Illes, J. (2013). Aging 2.0: health information about dementia on Twitter. *PLoS One 8* (7), e69861.

Rodriquez, J. (2013). 'Narrating dementia: self and community in an online forum.' *Qualitative Health Research 23* (9), 1215–1227.

Rohra, H. (2016). *Dementia Activist*. London: Mabuse Verlag.

Rosenberg, F., Parsa, A., Humble, L. and McGee, C. (2009). *Meet Me: Making Art Accessible to People with Dementia*. New York: MOMA.

Rossato-Bennett, Michael (dir.) (2014). *Alive Inside* [Film]. USA: Cadiz.

Rusted, J., Sheppard, L. and Waller, D. (2006). 'A multi-centre randomized control group trial on the use of art therapy for older people with dementia.' *Group Analysis 39* (4), 517–536.

Sabat, S. and Harré, R. (1992). 'The construction and deconstruction of self in Alzheimer's disease.' *Ageing and Society 12*, 443–461.

Selwood, A., Johnston, K., Katona, C., Lyketsos, C. and Livingston, G. (2007). 'Systematic review of the effect of psychological interventions on family caregivers of people with dementia.' *Journal of Affective Disorders 191* (1–3), 75–89.

Smith, R., Drennan, V., Mackenzie, A. and Greenwood, N. (2018). 'The impact of befriending and peer support on family carers of people living with dementia: a mixed methods study.' *Archives of Gerontology and Geriatrics 76*, 188–195.

Suchet, J. (2010). *My Bonnie*. London: Harper.

Swaffer, K. (2014). 'Reinvesting in life is the best prescription.' *Australian Journal of Dementia Care 3* (6), 31–32.

Swaffer, K. (2016). *What the Hell Happened to My Brain? Living Beyond Dementia*. London: Jessica Kingsley Publishers.

Swaffer, K. (2018). *Creating Life with Words, Love and Hope*. Accessed on 26/3/18 at https://kateswaffer.com/tag/phd.

Swaffer, K. (2019). *The Impact on Parents and Partners*. Accessed on 26/3/18 at www.youngdementiauk.org/impact-parents-partners.

Swinnen, A. (2016). 'Healing words: a study of poetry interventions in dementia care.' *Dementia 15* (6), 1377–1404.

Swinton, J. (2012). *Dementias: Living in the Memories of God*. Grand Rapids: Wm. B Eerdmans Publishing.

Takechi, H., Sugihara, Y., Matsumoto, H. and Yamada, H. (2018). 'A dementia café as a bridgehead for community-inclusive care: qualitative analysis of observations by on-the-job training participants in a dementia café.' *Dementia and Geriatric Cognitive Disorders 46* (3–4), 128–139.

Talbot, M. (2011). *Keeping Mum: Caring for Someone with Dementia*. London: Hay House.

Theurer, K.A. and Hall, J. (2016). It takes the loneliness away: Innovative peer support programming for dementia. Alzheimer's and Dementia. Conference: Alzheimer's Association International Conference 2016. Canada. 12 (7 Supplement), 790.

Unadkat, S., Camic, P.M. and Vella-Burrows, T. (2017). 'Understanding the experience of group singing for couples where one partner has a diagnosis of dementia.' *The Gerontologist 57* (3), 469–478.

Vella-Burrows, T. and Wilson, L. (2016). *Remember to Dance*. Accessed on 21/3/19 at www.canterbury.ac.uk/health-and-wellbeing/sidney-de-haan-research-centre/documents/remember-to-dance-summary-report.pdf.

Whitlatch, C., Judge, K., Zarit, S. and Femia, E. (2006). 'Dyadic intervention for family caregivers and care receivers in early-stage dementia.' *The Gerontologist 46* (5), 688–694.

Willis, E., Semple, A.C. and de Waal, H. (2018). 'Quantifying the benefits of peer support for people with dementia: a Social Return on Investment (SROI) study.' *Dementia 17* (3), 266–278.

World Alzheimer's Report (2018). *The State of the Art of Dementia Research: New Frontiers*. London: Alzheimer's Disease International.

Yalom, I. (2005). *Theory and Practice of Group Psychotherapy (5th Edition)*. New York: Basic Books.

Young Onset Dementia Support Group (n.d.). Accessed on 4/3/18 at www.facebook.com/YoungOnsetDementiaSupportPage.

Zeisel, J. (2008). *Art Therapy for Alzheimer's and Dementia*. Accessed on 17/5/19 at www.everydayhealth.com/alzheimers/webcasts/art-therapy-for-alzheimers-and-dementia-transcript-1.aspx.

Chapter 7

Dementia Champions

Introduction

As the title suggests, this chapter is all about *dementia champions* and some of the inspirational projects and initiatives that have been implemented. The concept of *champion* can be viewed as relating to individuals, groups, initiatives, resources, environmental modifications and societal innovations, all of which aim to improve the quality of life for those affected by dementia. Traditionally, views about dementia have tended towards pessimism as reflected by a number of narratives from both those diagnosed and family members regarding the receipt of a diagnosis as if it were a death sentence (Bryden 2018; Jackson 2010). It is a condition that is commonly related to *old people* and connected to concepts such as *senility*. There is an evident need to challenge assumptions and expectations that negatively impact upon individuals' lives, questioning the process of double discrimination, outlined by Morris and Morris (2010) as relating to the lowered expectations held on account of a person's advancing age or condition of dementia. A key message arising from the previous chapter concerned the importance of recognizing the person who still exists inside (and alongside) the condition of dementia and their capacity for new growth and future learning, as well as noting many ways in which people continued to live productive lives. This message continues to be promoted and championed by an increasing number of initiatives, projects and campaigns.

The story so far

The previous two chapters have shown us the spectrum of experiences that are represented by both states of struggling and coping. The focus upon coping provides a welcome counter to what is more commonly considered in terms of the dementia experience, namely loss, decline and pessimism. We have now seen how the Lawrence family are continuing with their lives, 'living beyond' Peter's diagnosis of dementia. A core resource for them is peer support and the many opportunities offered to feel connected with others who simply understand or 'get it'. They have also embraced ways and means for Peter to express himself and relieve feelings of tension through creative modes. The emphasis upon living beyond dementia highlights that people need not become defined totally by their diagnosis. Essentially, these all kindle feelings of optimism and help to promote personal autonomy.

Chapter themes

This chapter will introduce the reader to the following themes:

- personhood
- personhood and identity-affirming approaches
- projects, campaigns and innovations
- environmental initiatives
- media messages.

Personhood

Whilst there are merits in acknowledging the present endeavours in exploring and explaining dementia, one should also give a nod to earlier observers and commentators on the human psyche. The growing wave of positive energy permeating dementia care can be attributed to the foundation established by the pioneering Tom Kitwood and the Bradford Dementia Group (Kitwood 1997; Kitwood and Bredin 1992). Their studies and subsequent championing of personhood swept through dementia care facilities bringing a welcome breath of fresh air. Their reimagined approaches to care were an adaptation of humanistic philosophy and its intention of putting the client or patient first. This built upon the person-centred work of Carl Rogers (1961) and Abraham Maslow (1970) and was instrumental in the philosophical approach advocated within the national Dementia Care Strategy (Department of Health and Social Care 2009). Further adaptations and maintenance of this approach can be seen in the more recent work of Professor Murna Downs or Dr David Sheard (Dementia Care Matters). The humanistic movement in psychology supported the belief that humans, as individuals, are unique beings and should therefore be recognized and treated as such by psychiatrists and psychologists. This branch of psychology gained influence for its 'appreciation for the fundamental inviolability of the human experience' (Bugental 1963, p.563).

Humanistic principles and their application became popular in the US during the 1960s where humanists were concerned with the fullest growth of the individual in the areas of love, fulfilment, self-worth and autonomy. Abraham Maslow was a leading psychologist who wrote a seminal paper on motivation, diagrammatically portrayed as a pyramid. He describes needs as being arranged in a *hierarchy of pre-potency* and affirmed that when basic needs of a physiological nature and safety are met the individual can progress to higher levels such as belongingness and love, and esteem (Maslow 1943). The individual, on completion of these higher needs, can fully realize their potential through self-actualization. Maslow (1970, p.45) described esteem needs as one of the basic of human needs that contributed to the 'feeling of self-confidence, worth, strength, capacity, and adequacy, of being useful and necessary in the world'.

Carl Rogers (1946) postulated that for a person to 'grow' they needed an environment that provided them with genuineness (where there was openness and self-disclosure), acceptance (where the person was seen with unconditional positive regard) and empathy (where the person was being listened to and understood). Rogers (1967, p.34) contended that in order to show acceptance of the person then demonstrating respect was important: 'warm regard for him as a person of unconditional self-worth – of value no matter what his condition, his behaviour, or feelings'.

Rogers (1967, p.40) reasoned that a helping relationship had certain characteristics: 'a relationship in which at least one of the parties has the intent of promoting the growth, development, maturity, improved functioning, improved coping with life of the other'.

The influence of Rogerian thinking has been enormously influential upon the general way in which we construe therapeutic relationships and emotional difficulties. Some of these observations, commentaries and principles during the latter part of the twentieth century began to permeate into articles and research and be applied to dementia care. Within these publications and practices the focus upon 'the person with dementia' regarded the individual as central and their diagnosis as a secondary consideration. Doyle and Rubenstein (2014) argued that person-centred care represented a shift in focus away from the traditional biomedical approach towards a more holistic and individualized model. Furthermore the application of this approach stemmed from early theoretical work that demonstrated that a biomedical approach with a focus on mental pathology could compromise the personhood of people with dementia. Kitwood (1988) was an early critic who questioned the emphasis on individual neuropathology while important external factors on disease progression were overlooked. Whilst exploring the limitations of exclusively task orientated and authoritarian deficit focused care provision, Kitwood advocated the use of person-centredness in dementia care. Kitwood (1997) proposed that the biomedical orientation of many nursing aides fostered a narrow perspective, which did not fully consider the psychological, social and cultural complexities of the person with dementia. The restrictive and debilitating care approaches were recognised as *malignant social psychology* factors (Kitwood 1997) and detrimental to individuals' *marks of well-being* (Kitwood and Bredin 1992). This perspective prompted dementia caregivers to shift their focus towards the uniqueness of the *person*, placing this before their illness or disability. It emphasized the value in knowing the client, respecting their preferences and individual needs, working together through therapeutic interactions and facilitating a stimulating environment. To this end he began to develop person-centred guidance on communication and relationships with the person with dementia, challenging restrictive and negative attitudes and cultures in dementia care (Kitwood 1997).

Kitwood used the term 'person-centred care' to bring together ideas and ways of working that emphasized communication and relationships. He proposed that dementia could be best understood as interplay between neurological impairment and psycho-social factors, namely health, individual psychology and the environment, with particular emphasis on social context. He believed that the environment has as much effect on the brain as the brain has on a person's abilities (Kitwood 1998). Furthermore, Kitwood believed that the basic assumption in the medical sciences of dementia carried far too negative and predictable implications for the nature of caregiving.

Brooker (2003) proposed that in person-centred dementia care, the carer must value and respect the resident (or patient), regard all individuals with dementia as complete people, attempt to understand the experiences of the person with dementia and create a positive social environment. An extensive literature review by Kogan, Wilber and Mosquedo (2016) for definitions of person-centred care identified 15 definitions that addressed 17 principles or values. The review found that the six most prominent domains involved person-centred care holistic care, choice, respect and value, dignity, self-determination and purposeful living.

The findings suggested that it was clear that there is a shift in focus away from a traditional biomedical model in favour of embracing personal choice and autonomy.

ACTIVITY 7.1

When did you first come across the term 'personhood', what was the context and what was your initial understanding?

Why do you think personhood appears so prominently in dementia care literature?

From a practitioner perspective, does the term 'personhood' or its underlying philosophy appear in your working practices and, if so, how is it demonstrated?

A consequence of past pejorative attitudes can be problematic in the present as we may retain from personal experience or through conversations with others a negative and pessimistic view of dementia. Changing minds may require more than a 'positive spin' or memorable tag line. And yet encouraging conversations that both seek to reduce stigma and increase understanding of dementia and empowering people with dementia are so important. Figure 7.1 presents the reader with two points in time when dementia has been in the political spotlight. Both reports provide a minimal interpretation and further reading is recommended. But the themes are replicating both concerns and strategies, and arguably are seeking to change or challenge views about dementia and the services provided.

The increase in the number of people diagnosed and the drive to raise awareness about the dementia experience (Department of Health and Social Care 2009) is marked by a greater societal visibility of this condition. There are now more people sharing their experiences, aided by prominent figures and role models such as the celebrated Discworld author Sir Terry Pratchett, former American President Ronald Reagan and the famous country music singer Glen Campbell. Their personal expressions have had a beneficial and inspirational impact, assisting others in appreciating what is encountered first-hand and raising awareness of what their support needs include. Terry Pratchett became an Alzheimer's Society ambassador, giving talks, fronting television documentaries and promoting the Out of the Shadows project (Alzheimer's Society 2008).

Living Well with Dementia (Department of Health and Social Care 2009)		*The Prime Minister's Challenge on Dementia 2020 (2015)*
• Raising awareness of dementia • Removing the stigma surrounding the condition • Improving diagnostic rates • Increasing the range of services for people with dementia and their carers	Changing our minds may be the first step in becoming a CHAMPION	• Boosting research • Improving care • Raising awareness • Implementation Plan (2016) • Risk reduction • Health and care • Awareness and social action research

Figure 7.1 Dementia reports

Ronald Reagan's (1994) letter to the nation reported upon his dementia diagnosis:

> We feel it is important to share it with you. In opening our hearts, we hope this might promote greater awareness of this condition. Perhaps it will encourage a clearer understanding of the individuals and families who are affected by it.

This heartfelt letter promoted dialogue and awareness-raising around the dementia experience.

The documentary film *Glen Campbell: I'll Be Me* made public the singer's Alzheimer's diagnosis and showed how it affected his performances during his final musical tour. This critically acclaimed film was one of the few films achieving a 100 per cent rating on Rotten Tomatoes, a review website for television programmes and films. The reviews were testament to the inspiration derived from this film: 'Alzheimer's is such a sad disease but they seem to make it uplifting somehow.'

What such role models do is to aid in challenging stigmatizing societal attitudes, placing greater emphasis and focus upon the person over and above that of the condition of dementia and related symptoms. This chapter and the previous one highlight such examples and the promotion amongst those with dementia and their families of the crucial element of *hope*. The energy and collective support for dementia promotion can be seen within memorable straplines (Walking for Dementia) and soubriquets (Dementia Champions) that appear to have become a mantra for encouraging our understanding about dementia and promoting fundraising. Arguably, this type of campaigning seeks to lift the lid on often long-held social views and cultural taboos surrounding dementia and the people who have this diagnosis.

Personhood and identity-affirming approaches

Fazio *et al.* (2018) identified a number of recommendations for implementing person-centred care, which included better understanding the person with dementia and their personal values, beliefs, likes and dislikes; appreciating the person's perceptual reality; facilitating and promoting opportunities for meaningful engagement; fostering a supportive milieu for individuals, families and staff; aiding effective caring relationships; and regularly evaluating care, making required changes.

Examples of these will be examined within this section, reflecting upon some of the approaches and interventions utilized in the affirmation of the personhood of those affected through dementia, namely reminiscence and validation.

Reminiscence

A core identity-reaffirming intervention involves the process of reconnecting with events, experiences and feelings that resonate strongly for individuals and family members. This involves the approach of reminiscence, a term that can be defined as:

- a story told about a past event remembered by the narrator
- the enjoyable recollection of past events.

(Oxford English Dictionary 2020)

This definition picks up on two key elements. First, the narrative involved that contextualizes experiences and recalled stimuli. Second, the affirmation that there can be a sense of pleasure and enhanced well-being. As a therapeutic intervention, reminiscence engages a biographical process using stimuli such as music or pictures where the past can be recalled. It has been defined as a vocal or silent recall of events in a person's life, either alone or with another person or groups of people (Spector *et al.* 2004; Woods *et al.* 1992). It originates in Butler's (1963) work on *life review* in which past experience and unresolved conflicts are brought into consciousness. Closely related to reminiscence therapy, life story work focuses upon putting together a life story album for an individual (Moos and Bjorn 2006). The aims of reminiscence therapy and life story work are varied and include:

- uncovering or preserving individual identity (Murphy 2000; Clarke, Hanson and Ross 2003)

- improving the quality of life through the impact of 'being listened to' (McKee *et al.* 2003)
- allowing healthcare staff to see beyond a person's diagnosis (Murphy 2000; Clarke *et al.* 2003)
- facilitating communication between the person with dementia and their families (Batson, Thorne and Peak 2002)
- providing enjoyment (Murphy 2000).

These benefits outline positive outcomes not only for the person with dementia but also for family members and healthcare personnel. Evidence suggests that reminiscence therapy can lead to overall improvements in depression and loneliness and promote psychological well-being (Chiang *et al.* 2010). A study by McKee *et al.* (2003) identified several positive effects of reminiscence therapy and emphasized the enjoyment and engagement of those involved. The Alzheimer's Society is strongly in favour of the reminiscence therapy approach as outlined in their publication *Memories are Made of This* (Heathcote 2009).

The dementia charity Memory Box Network highlights four key content types that therapists can use to help connect an individual's surroundings to years gone by:

- written material
- audio files
- still images
- moving images.

This illustrates some of the ways in which memories can be stimulated utilizing audio-visual channels. Clearly, the type of stimuli can be broadened to also encompass some very vibrant recollections through smell, taste and touch. An important element to consider is how reminiscence activities are approached and it would seem more appropriate to offer stimuli as an invitation for responding, rather than posing the question 'Do you remember?', with its obvious limitations.

As Gibson (2004) asserts, research on reminiscence has tended to focus on outcomes for persons with dementia but we also need to look at the impact on carers and family members to fully appreciate its value. There are important relationship benefits in the present time between people with dementia and their carers through their involvement in reminiscence therapy (Clarke *et al.* 2003; McKeown, Clarke and Repper 2006; Schweitzer and Bruce 2008; Woods *et al.* 2009). An essential dynamic operating between the person with dementia and their partner is the coming together and reinforcement of their identity as a couple. This benefit can be extended to healthcare staff who have reported warmer feelings and better understanding of those with dementia when having knowledge of their life histories (Pietrukowicz and Johnson 1991).

The TV series *Dementiaville* (Channel 4 2015) illustrated how shared experiences from past times can be re-engaged in by family members with powerful benefits for all concerned. In this programme we see various examples of families reconnecting with each other, doing things that were regarded as part of the family's collective identity. For example, two sons recollect that they used to go camping as a family, an activity that was subsequently greatly missed. We later see the whole family (person with dementia included) quietly sitting next to their tent eating a meal and enjoying the tranquillity of the evening. This illustrates a process of collective reminiscence in relation to past experiences that resonate powerfully for all members. It extends the concept of reminiscence to acknowledge that reinforced identity applies equally to couples and family groups as well as to individuals.

ACTIVITY 7.2

If I had dementia, which might be a difficult question to respond to, what unique aspects *about myself* would it be important that others should know?

You may want to develop your response by considering the following:

- hobbies and interests
- life experiences
- personal and professional achievements
- likes and dislikes
- occupations
- personal characteristics.

From a practitioner perspective, what practices do you use to discover 'who the person is' and identify the benefits this can have for developing an awareness and understanding of their life?

The next part of this section introduces the reader to a selection of reminiscence projects.

FOOTBALL MEMORIES

This project united participants around their shared passion for and interest in football. It demonstrated changes in mood, behaviour and levels of engagement in many of the men who participated and was regarded as inspirational by care staff and family members. Indeed as stated by one participant's partner: 'I drive here with this sad person with dementia and I take home my husband.'

In these reminiscence groups many men found themselves taking centre stage, reeling off expert knowledge and sharing collective memories, which brought laughter and camaraderie to the group and a boost to their self-esteem (Schofield and Tolson 2010). (www.footballmemories.org.uk/content/the_project)

REMEMBERING YESTERDAY CARING TODAY

This intervention involves people with dementia and family carers together. It includes a structured programme for exploring their lived past life together in the present. Activities involve artistic expression, drawing, dramatic improvisations singing and dance. It was noted that even people who were unable to articulate verbally enjoyed joining in vicariously. (www.storiedlives.institute/remembering-yesterday-caring-today)

LET'S TALK ABOUT DEMENTIA

This project has been run across a number of care homes and introduced a series of discussion topics. It utilizes pictures and memorabilia to stimulate recall. (https://letstalkaboutdementia.wordpress.com/2015/01/29/8-amazing-stories-from-the-reminiscence-projects)

LET'S CHAT

The Alzheimer's Society's (2018) *Dementia Together* showcases an initiative created by Taruna, drawing upon her Hindu Indian background to create a set of cards called Let's Chat, prompting memories around food, travel, clothes and religion for people from South Asian communities. (www.alzheimers.org.uk/dementia-together-magazine/june-july-2018/lets-chat-reminiscence-cards-draw-south-asian-experiences)

BBC REMARC

The BBC Reminiscence Archive is designed to trigger memories and reminiscence in people with dementia. The most frequently chosen decades are the 1940s, 1950s and 1960s with the most popular themes being People, Events, Music, Sport, TV and Radio. These resources were positively engaged with by participants. (www.bbc.co.uk/rd/blog/2017-02-bbc-rem-arc-dementia-memories-archive)

THE EUROPEAN REMINISCENCE NETWORK

The European Reminiscence Network aims to promote best practice in reminiscence work and to share experience across national boundaries. It has facilitated the development of a series of international projects with some being widely cited within publications. (www.europeanreminiscencenetwork.org)

HOUSE OF MEMORIES

The House of Memories is a museum-led reminiscence programme. They provide access to a selection of museum objects, activities and associated resources to facilitate sharing of memories and experience. (https://houseofmemories.co.uk)

GUIDED REMINISCENCE – ALIVE

This project utilizes images, music and multi-sensory objects to encourage conversation and promote reconnection with personal interests. It incorporates a number of technological resources including iPads to engage individuals with topics and themes of relevance for them. (https://aliveactivities.org/alive/en/activity-sessions/guided-reminiscence)

MUSEUM OF LAKELAND LIFE AND INDUSTRY

This museum has a collection of over 5000 photos of daily life from the Lake District, Cumbria. These photographs were taken between the 1930s and 1960s by Joseph Hardman and are regularly used as reminiscence aids for people with dementia. (www.lakelandmuseum.org.uk)

* * *

This is only a small number of the projects and initiatives being offered and essentially we are only restricted by the confines of our own imagination with numerous available resources and aids to utilize. For example, YouTube offers a wealth of videos spanning many decades and should have something of interest for everyone. Similarly, images and photos can be easily accessed from a wide range of internet sites, for example, Getty images. Further resources can be found in local libraries, museums, clubs and organizations. Bradford's National Media Museum in West Yorkshire, England, for example, has numerous pictures and objects to spark interest and discussion along with their video viewing resource TV Heaven where programmes spanning decades can be watched.

ACTIVITY 7.3

Think of a piece of music, a photograph, a book and a TV programme that entertained you during your youth.

Now as an adult, when presented with one or all of the above, what memories and feelings do they engender?

Do you find yourself reminiscing more the older you become?

From a practitioner perspective, do you encourage reminiscence approaches with the person and if so why? If you do, provide examples. If not, what could you offer?

Validation therapy

The essence of *validation therapy*, developed by Naomi Feil in the 1960s and 1970s, concerns connection and engagement with those experiencing dementia. Its core principle relates to the communicating to another person that they are acknowledged, respected, listened to and, regardless of whether or not the listener actually agrees with the content, treated with genuine respect, rather than being marginalized or dismissed (Feil 2013; Feil 2014). What this means in essence is that we genuinely form a connection with others who in turn feel properly *heard* by us. It is in sharp contrast to the approach of Reality Orientation (RO), which was heavily promoted across dementia care services some decades ago. A strong criticism of RO was that people living with dementia were constantly being contradicted and 're-educated' in order to be brought to the shared reality of practitioners or carers. Further arguments reflected upon it 'being applied in a mechanical, inflexible, insensitive and confrontational manner' (Woods *et al.* 2012, p.3).

It does indeed appear to be somewhat harsh and uncaring with its seeming preoccupation upon a person's deficits in memory and cognition, highlighting more what a person *can't do* as opposed to what they *can do*. This is where validation differs, providing a polarized opposite with its emphasis upon appreciating and validating the reality of another's emotional experience. The actor Christopher Eccleston (*The Guardian* 2015), talking about his father's experience, reflected: 'Dementia dismantled my father's personality... I eventually learned that, instead of trying to pull people with dementia into your world, you have to enter theirs.'

The statement 'you have to enter their [world]' expresses very succinctly the importance for health carers in being mindful of the perceptual reality as experienced by those with dementia. It also encapsulates Christine Bryden's (2005) concept of 'dancing with dementia', matching our movement to that of the other person. Essentially, the validation approach is about respect, enabling individuals to feel heard and acknowledged for what *they* are experiencing and feeling. An issue perhaps of contention relating to validation involves that of truth telling. Information provided by the Alzheimer's Society (2019a) for carers to consider includes:

- Is there a message behind the question that indicates an emotion or unmet need, for example, fear, loneliness or disorientation?
- Is the person likely to understand what they are being told? Are there ways of making it easier for them to understand?
- Would knowing the truth cause the person significant distress? If so, would the consequences of telling the truth outweigh the need?
- Are there ways of telling the person the truth that would be less upsetting?
- Are there some things that are essential to be honest about?
- Will not telling the truth make things more difficult in the long run?
- From your knowledge of the person, what do you think they would want?

For the past two decades, David Sheard (Founder of Dementia Care Matters) and his team have been paving the way for modern dementia care with their Feelings Matter Most approach and the Butterfly Model. He has a strong track record of inspiring and leading change, focusing firmly upon the person with dementia and their essential sense of self. His work was featured in the BBC (2009) TV documentaries *Can Gerry Robinson Fix Dementia Care Homes?* and *Dementiaville*, which championed the validity and worth of those with dementia. David Sheard's Butterfly Household Model of Care allows persons with dementia to believe they are working, getting married or having a family again, something he defends as a potent and caring method for reducing distress for those with dementia and their families. This is supported by Rudgard who states:

> If you're a family member, you have two choices. Either all your time spent with them you're trying to force them to remember events, or you accept the person as they are, you accept that you can't fix them because of the brain damage, and you learn to love them in their new reality. (*The Telegraph* 2015)

This embracing of a person's *new reality* can be regarded as both supportive and caring with individuals feeling acknowledged and in connection with others.

Working through this section, you will have noted a challenge to the traditional view, which sees the identity and personality of those with dementia gradually disappearing. We can reframe this and instead note problems with communication and cognition that impede expression or recognition of self. There are a variety of innovative and engaging approaches being used, including reminiscence and validation, to reach out and connect with people with dementia. This provides them with a vibrant and potent means of self-expression. In some instances the results can be transformative with individuals apparently 'reawakening' and reconnecting with self and their external environment. The impact is also felt by carers with opportunities to re-engage with partners.

Projects, campaigns and innovations

The previous two decades have witnessed an increased media-driven awareness of dementia and its impact on the person, carers, significant people in their life and the wider community, be it from a local, national or global perspective. In the spirit of promoting awareness it appears marketing strategies embrace our cognisance of dementia, providing we find the time to accept these messages or, if necessary, wish to challenge our preconceived pejorative attitudes.

Arguably, campaigning seeks to challenge often long-held social views and cultural taboos surrounding dementia. Changing attitudes may be the first step to making all of us champions. A winning start would be to encourage conversations that both seek to reduce stigma and increase understanding. This section features a range of recent projects, campaigns and initiatives aimed at championing the experience of those affected by dementia. Please note, given the steady development of related work, the selection of work shown here is not intended to be definitive and it is to be expected that many wonderful projects will not be covered here.

ACTIVITY 7.4

What type of professional journals, research articles and media sources have you recently read about dementia?

What has caught your attention, for example, headlines, medical optimism, sensationalism, marketing and advertising? Have these messages been positive or not?

From a practitioner perspective, what local or national reporting of dementia would you wish to see and where?

Examples of projects, campaigns and innovations

IDEAL

The University of Exeter's IDEAL programme (2014–2022) explores people's experiences of living well with dementia. It involves over 1540 people with dementia and 1280 carers exploring factors helping them to live well. (www.idealproject.org.uk)

DEMENTIA 4 SCHOOLS (INTERGENERATIONAL SCHOOLS PROJECT)

This collaborative initiative (2012–2013) engaged 21 schools in a pioneer project offering a diverse range of teaching resources and events to teach children about dementia. Over 2000 children participated in activities including dementia awareness lessons, choir visits to dementia care homes, debates and art, drama and music projects. This project was followed by the Alzheimer's Society's Youth Engagement project. (www.dementiaaction.org.uk/dementiafriendlyschools/dementia_4_schools_project)

DEMENTIA DIARIES

The UK Dementia Diaries project collects people's diverse experiences of living with dementia within a series of audio diaries. It provides a public record and personal archive documenting narratives of daily lives of people living with dementia. The aim of this initiative is to prompt dialogue and change attitudes concerning the experience of dementia. (https://dementiadiaries.org)

DEMENTIA ENGAGEMENT AND EMPOWERMENT PROJECT (DEEP)

DEEP is a UK network consisting of around 100 groups of people with dementia. These groups are strongly rooted in their local communities, including some in care homes. It records members' views about issues important to them. They are also involved in producing guides that share good practice and learning. It is a 'rights-based' organization encouraging groups to identify and speak out about the issues that are important to *them* (not just 'consulted' about issues that are important to *others*). (www.dementiavoices.org.uk)

PRIDE IN CARE

Pride in Care concerns a quality standard for organizations to show how they support LGBT+ people. (www.alzheimers.org.uk/dementia-together-magazine-dec-19jan-20/pride-care-promoting-inclusivity-and-understanding)

BRING DEMENTIA OUT

Bring Dementia Out is an Alzheimer's Society project to encourage dementia awareness and inclusion in Brighton and Manchester, UK. (www.alzheimers.org.uk/dementia-professionals/dementia-experience-toolkit/real-life-examples/supporting-inclusion/lgbt-inclusion-brighton-manchester)

EARLY STAGE DEMENTIA PROJECT

Age Scotland's Early Dementia Project seeks to raise awareness of early-stage dementia and the signs and symptoms of the condition. This project incorporates information and advice, runs dementia awareness workshops and promotes inclusive communities. (www.ageuk.org.uk/scotland/what-we-do/dementia/age-scotlands-early-stage-dementia-project)

THE MACINTYRE DEMENTIA PROJECT (2016)

The MacIntyre Dementia Special Interest Group (DSIG) received a significant grant from the Department of Health's Innovation, Excellence and Strategic Development Fund to create a range of learning and multi-media information resources to improve the support and care for people with learning disabilities who have dementia or are at risk of developing dementia. (www.macintyrecharity.org/our-expertise/dementia/the-macintyre-dementia-project)

STRENGTHENING RESPONSES TO DEMENTIA IN DEVELOPING COUNTRIES (STRIDE)

The London School of Economics and Political Science's STRiDE programme examines economics, epidemiology and policy analyses to determine responses to the needs of those affected by dementia in an ethical and sustainable way. It aims to increase dementia awareness and reduce stigma for families living with dementia. (www.lse.ac.uk/pssru/research/projects/dementia/STRiDE)

FROM SELDOM HEARD TO SEEN AND HEARD

In 2017, the National Dementia Action Alliance launched 'From Seldom Heard to Seen and Heard', a campaign aimed at improving outcomes for people living with dementia and their carers in groups who are often overlooked such as:

- LGBT
- prison population
- people with learning disabilities.

(www.dementiaaction.org.uk/joint_work/dementia_and_seldom_heard_groups)

EUROPEAN PREVENTION OF ALZHEIMER'S DEMENTIA CONSORTIUM (EPAD)

The EPAD is an interdisciplinary research programme spanning public and private sector organizations across Europe. They are committed to increasing understanding about Alzheimer's dementia and approaches for preventing and treating it. (http://ep-ad.org)

MEMORY WALK

Memory Walk is a sponsored walk for all ages and abilities. The walks are spread across England, Wales and Northern Ireland, routed through either a city, woodlands or park. (https://www.memorywalk.org.uk)

GLOBAL DEMENTIA ACTION PLAN

The World Health Organization's Global Action Plan aims to improve the lives of people with dementia, their carers and families, as well as decreasing the impact of dementia on communities and countries. (www.who.int/mental_health/neurology/dementia/action_plan_2017_2025/en)

PLAYLIST FOR LIFE

Playlist for Life is about the power of music and the strong connection people form with music. This charity's intentions are for each person with dementia to have their own unique and personal playlist that reflects and reinforces their life story. (www.playlistforlife.org.uk)

SPORTING MEMORIES

The Sporting Memories Foundation and football chiefs have collaborated upon a project that aims to support former players diagnosed with dementia. This offers advice regarding day-to-day living as well as financial and legal aspects. (www.sportingmemoriesnetwork.com/news/pfa-practical-guide-to-living-with-dementia)

BAT: BOUNCE FOR ALZHEIMER'S

The BAT Foundation offer enjoyment, social contact, physical exercise and a welcome diversion for those with dementia through playing table tennis. Their specially designed table and equipment facilitates the playing experience. (www.batfoundation.com)

DEMENTIA ADVENTURE

Dementia Adventure specialize in designing and delivering small-group short breaks and holidays for people living with dementia, their partners, family, friends or carer to enjoy together. (www.dementiaadventure.co.uk)

MERI YAADAIN

The Bradford-based Meri Yaadain ('my memories') initiative provides timely support for the South Asian community. Their support is targeted towards families and organizations involved in dementia care. They also provide a service of awareness-raising. (www.meriyaadain.co.uk)

HEALTH AND WELL-BEING ALLIANCE PROJECT

This UK project targets black, Asian and minority ethnic communities affected by dementia. It sets out five key areas involving partnership, resources, professional events, community events and research engagement. (Jeraj and Butt 2018)

SOMALI MENTAL HEALTH NETWORK/ BANGLADESHI MENTAL HEALTH NETWORK

These networks are based in Camden, London and were developed to attend to the lack of awareness of dementia in the BAME communities. Through the networks, information and best practice are shared and ensuing discussions help to ensure services are tailored to meet the needs of these communities. (www.alzheimers.org.uk/sites/default/files/migrate/downloads/appg_2013_bame_report.pdf)

SIDE BY SIDE

The Side by Side initiative is aimed at supporting individuals through one-to-one engagement to involve themselves in activities that are meaningful to them. (https://www.alzheimers.org.uk/get-support/your-support-services/side-by-side)

DEMENTIA DEKH BHAAL (TO CARE FOR DEMENTIA)

This project supports South Asian carers of people with dementia in Rochdale, UK. (www.tide.uk.net/dementia-dekh-baal-evaluation-report)

TIDE

The Tide project aims to support carers of people with dementia to express their needs. This involves creating partnerships with care organizations. (www.tide.uk.net)

EVERY THIRD MINUTE FESTIVAL

Every Third Minute, a festival of theatre, dementia and hope, is a unique collaboration between nine festival curators (people living with dementia, their family and friends) and theatre-makers at Leeds Playhouse. Over 7500 attended events, including the stage adaptation of Lisa Genova's *Still Alice*, which was guided by the activist Wendy Mitchell. (https://leedsplayhouse.org.uk/events/every-third-minute)

INNOVATIONS IN DEMENTIA

Innovations in Dementia is a community interest company working nationally with people with dementia, partner organizations and professionals with the clear aim of developing and testing projects that have the potential for enhancing the lives of people with dementia. (www.innovationsindementia.org.uk)

Environmental initiatives

The environmental culture can be difficult to change; as illustrated so vividly within the TV documentary *Can Gerry Robinson Fix Dementia Care Homes?*, it relies upon effective leadership. An example of some of the intractability concerning staff opposition to making the environmental setting more homely included voiced concerns that residents 'might eat the plants'. This was challenged by Dr David Sheard asking the question 'Is it OK though to kill people with boredom?' The illustration here shows the importance of reframing and questioning attitudinal obstacles and promoting fresh ways of reaffirming personal identity, providing stimulation and comfort as well as attending to a person's overall well-being. This section therefore examines the potency and value to those with dementia and their families from attending to the environment within which they live.

Dementia Friends

The Dementia Friends campaign, spearheaded by the Alzheimer's Society, is concerned with the environment from a broader perspective. It is a major initiative aimed at challenging discriminatory attitudes and awareness-raising, engaging individuals, groups, local businesses and organizations (e.g. Lewisham and Greenwich NHS Trust; Marks and Spencer (M&S); Lloyd's Banking Group). The organizations getting involved offer dementia-awareness training for their staff members. M&S, for example, launched this initiative in 2014 with all 79,600 staff members becoming Dementia Friends. The benefits of such initiatives to those living with dementia will be clearly apparent.

ACTIVITY 7.5

Within your community where, how and by whom have dementia-friendly initiatives been established?

Have you frequented any of these initiatives?

From a practitioner perspective, does the organization/service you work for support any community-based initiatives?

Is there a need for health or social care involvement?

There are many variations of Dementia Friends being attached to activities and local events such as:

- dementia-friendly swimming
- dementia-friendly theatre performances (e.g. West Yorkshire Playhouse)
- dementia-friendly cinema screenings.

The Alzheimer's Society offers guidance for such organizations to create dementia-friendly experiences within their venues. The cinema guide, for example, created in partnership with the UK Cinema Association and the British Film Institute's Film Audience Network, contains practical advice concerning safety, comfort and tips for promotion and programme scheduling.

> For a person living with dementia, watching a film in the cinema has many benefits. It can promote activity and stimulation of the mind, can be an important tool of reminiscence, and is associated with relaxation, engagement and, above all, enjoyment. (Alzheimer's Society 2017)

These important elements can also be complemented by enhanced feelings of 'normality', the maintenance of one's social life.

Whilst laudable, dementia-friendly organizations need to ensure that training and awareness-raising is maintained. Ken Clasper (2014) praises initiatives engaging companies and communities; however, he urges: 'I know that many bus companies claim to have had their staff trained to support people with dementia, yet many are very rude when asked simple questions' (Clasper 2014).

> Over the last few years, a lot of work has been done in banks to make them Dementia Friendly, but I do wonder if they have now had second thoughts… These days the staff in our local branch insist on pushing people to use the machines, rather than speaking to a person at the till… It worries me that many other companies are claiming to be Dementia Friendly…but not actually following through and doing something positive for those living with dementia. (Clasper 2017)

Ken Clasper's comments show the importance of attending to dementia-friendly initiatives and ensuring that they continue to work effectively for those concerned.

Dementia-friendly communities

Dementia-friendly communities seek to address the targets outlined by the Prime Minister's Challenge on Dementia 2020 by creating communities around the UK that make a person with dementia's daily living and activities more accessible. The concept of 'dementia-friendly communities' has been interpreted in the UK in a number of ways. First, as previously mentioned, one of the policy initiatives outlined in the Prime Minister's Challenge on Dementia, is encouraging cities, towns and villages to sign up to become more dementia friendly. Second, the Alzheimer's Society 'Dementia-Friendly

Communities' programme encourages and facilitates the development of these communities. Third, cities, towns and villages can become publicly recognized for their work towards the Alzheimer's Society programme on dementia-friendly communities. There does not appear to be a standard model or template for the development of dementia-friendly communities; however, some research groups have identified foundations that could promote the establishment of such communities. An example by Crampton, Dean and Eley (2012), a 'four cornerstones' model, outlined creating a dementia-friendly York, in North Yorkshire. The four cornerstones are:

- *Place* – how does the physical environment, housing, neighbourhood and transport support the person with dementia?
- *People* – how do carers, families, friends, neighbours, health and social care professionals, especially general physicians, and the wider community respond to and support the person with dementia?
- *Resources* – are there sufficient services and facilities that are appropriate and supportive of the person with dementia? How well can people use the ordinary resources of the community?
- *Networks* – do those who support the person with dementia communicate, collaborate and plan together sufficiently well to provide the best support and to use people's own 'assets' well?

Alzheimer's Disease International (2016) suggested a similar model with a more proactive approach in actively involving people with dementia in all the stages of the community development. In this model the four cornerstones are:

- *people* (involvement of people with dementia)
- *communities* (the social and physical environments)
- *organizations* (dementia-friendly organizations and access to appropriate healthcare bodies)
- *partnerships* (cross-sectional support, collective commitment and collaboration of organizations).

These all-encompassing models illustrate the depth and variety of elements involved and requiring attention.

Dementia Adventure

In 2009 a social enterprise called Dementia Adventure was established to offer holiday breaks for people living with dementia and their carers. It also provides training and support to organizations. Natural England highlighted how engagement with nature and the great outdoors could be improved for the benefit of people living with dementia and their carers (Mapes *et al.* 2016). The project set out to obtain the views of 50–60 people living with dementia and 100–125 family carers in order to highlight what motivates people, what the barriers are and how they can be overcome to improve access and maximize the benefits this can bring to people. This was a collaborative project between Natural England, Dementia Adventure, Mental Health Foundation and Innovations in Dementia to inform the design of a large-scale demonstration project that will deliver services in the natural environment for people living with dementia and their carers. This report follows on from the *Greening Dementia* report (Clarke *et al.* 2013), which recommended large-scale research and evaluation studies to more robustly quantify the benefits of engaging with nature for people living with dementia, particularly with regard to the mental and physical health benefits and the cost benefits of different intervention types involving nature against more traditional medical treatments. The summary highlights the key findings from both people living with dementia and carers:

ACTIVITIES

- *Informal walking* was the most commonly cited activity. Several carers talked about the calming effect that this had on the person they cared for and it was an activity engaged in at least several times a week. It was also noted as vitally important as an escape from the pressures of being indoors, and was regarded as being as important to the carer as to the person with dementia.
- *Wildlife watching*, usually bird watching, is very popular amongst people living with dementia with positive effects received from their encounters with wildlife.

PLACES

- *Locations associated with water* (inland, coast, natural, artificial) were the most popular places to visit with canals, waterways, seaside, beach and coastal areas accessed at least once a month. Lakes in particular were positively regarded as environments where the person living with dementia and their carer could relax.
- *City parks or public gardens* were also popular among people with dementia, visited at least once a month. Several people with dementia

talked passionately about the role their local park played in providing them with somewhere to go, and as somewhere to enjoy watching other people taking part in activities.

The most important factors for both people with dementia and carers, helping or hindering their engagement with nature, were transport and mobility, availability, 'someone to take me', or personal attributes (limited physical mobility).

The care environment

The dementia-friendly initiatives recounted above are geared towards helping individuals feel safe, reassured, engaged and connected. Such initiatives are complemented by approaches offering modifications or additions to a person's environmental setting, which champion independence as well as being identity reaffirming. This is of vital importance for those experiencing changes in cognition and functioning to promote autonomy and maintenance of personhood. The following examples showcase some of the innovations being offered.

ARCHITECTURE

To begin with, we can consider the structure and layout of buildings and how they can enhance the well-being and comfort of those with dementia. A key starting point involves the design of homely rather than institutional or special care buildings. Related examples are illustrated by the University of Stirling regarding buildings with 'ordinary' tenement-like exterior appearance, common to the part of Scotland they are sited within (Turpie 2017). There are some important characteristics in terms of buildings' interiors for architects to be mindful of, including lighting and acoustics. McNair, Cunningham and Pollock (2010) identify features promoting visual comfort and orientation and suggest:

- Increase light levels to twice 'normal'.
- Use daylight where possible.
- Expose people to 24-hour cycle of light and dark.
- Use sufficient domestic style fittings to promote recognition of place.
- Include porches, gazebos and conservatories.
- Use contrasts in tone to aid perception of surfaces and objects, for example, food from plates.
- Attend to joins in floor covering that could be perceived as steps.

Attending to the acoustic design of buildings is needed because of the potential 'nuisance' factor impacting upon comfort, causing distractions and posing difficulties for communication. Building design should therefore aim to reduce background noise (e.g. from traffic); include greater areas of absorptive surfaces in larger living spaces; include acoustical separation between rooms; and show consideration to reverberation time from architectural surfaces, which could cause speech and sounds to be heard as an echo (Pollock 2014b). Outdoor spaces are also meaningful, with focus needed upon areas that are relaxing, bright and sunny as well as having available shade and shelter from the wind and noise. The environment should feel safe and secure with barrier-free access provided with level and non-slip surfacing, no sharply contrasting colours in surfacing or door threshold that could be seen as steps (Pollock 2014a).

HOGEWEYK

If we reflect upon the residential environment there are some striking examples challenging the detrimental factors identified within Kitwood's (1997) *malignant social psychology*. Leading the way, Hogeweyk (part of the Hogewey care centre) is a Dutch pioneering project with a village setting as the environment for residents with dementia to live in. According to Yvonne van Amerongen, one of the co-founders, Hogewey started out as an ordinary care home where: 'people sat watching TV, doing nothing, waiting for medication, for meals... It wasn't living. It was a kind of dying.'

However, the transformation of the care setting resulted in residents appearing alert, engaged and happy, spending their days in a more natural fashion, shopping, getting their hair done or going to the pub (Fernandes 2012). This is complemented by the ethos of care staff at Hogeweyk who are trained to focus on highlighting what residents can do as opposed to what they can't (Weller 2017).

MEADOW VIEW

Meadow View, a specialist dementia residential care centre, takes on board all the latest design for dementia research. It is a collaborative development between the Royal Institute of British Architects (RIBA) and the Dementia Services Development Centre at the University of Stirling. The design features centre around management, layout, interior design, landscaping and lighting that aim at creating a *home* as opposed to an *institution*. The layout is designed to aid the visitors' and residents' ability to navigate around the building with visual clues offered and access and activity areas carefully arranged to avoid creating confusion or frustration. Natural daylight is maximized, with large windows in key spaces (RIBA 2017).

ALEXA NURSING HOME

The Alexa Nursing Home in Germany facilitates the triggering of memories by re-creating settings from the East German communist era as a form of reminiscence therapy. They have a 'memory room' stocked with items commonly used in 1960s communist East Germany including old radios, passports, hair dryers and widely known ice cream advertisements (Noack 2017).

BENRATH SENIOR CENTRE

Benrath Senior Centre in Düsseldorf, Germany installed an exact replica of a standard bus stop outside. They found errant residents waiting at the bus stop, before forgetting why they were there. Richard Neureither, Benrath's director, stated: 'We will approach them and say that the bus is coming later and invite them in for a coffee' (*The Telegraph* 2008).

* * *

The settings and architectural considerations covered above show some of the current thinking about the living space of those affected by dementia. Good design aids well-being, lowers confusion and aids in feelings of safety, security and comfort. Allied to these factors are the burgeoning range of technological resources and approaches being developed to maximize independent living within one's living area, which will be covered next.

Assistive Technology (Telecare)

There are many examples of assistive technology with new products and services being added on a continuous basis. As defined by the Alzheimer's Society:

> Assistive technology refers to devices or systems that support a person to maintain or improve their independence, safety and wellbeing. It tends to refer to devices and systems that assist people with memory problems or other cognitive difficulties, rather than those that are used to aid someone with mobility or physical difficulties. (Alzheimer's Society 2019b)

A list of product types is given below:

DAILY LIVING

- automated prompts and reminders
- clocks and calendars
- medication aids
- automatic dispensers for pills
- locator devices and solutions
- communication aids
- talking mats.

SAFETY

- automatic lights that come on when the person is moving around
- automated shut-off devices, for example, gas
- water isolation devices (to turn off a tap if it's left running, preventing flooding)
- special plugs for water depth
- water heat sensor
- fall sensors
- telephone blockers that can be used to stop nuisance calls
- safer walking
- an alarm system – providing an alert when someone has moved outside a set boundary
- tracking devices or location monitoring services.

(Alzheimer's Society 2019b)

The range and scope of technological aids is developing at a rapid rate with some surprising and intriguing examples noted. For example, the Shintomi Nursing Home in Tokyo, Japan has over 20 models of care robots, mimicking cute furry animals, small children, human-shaped 'humanoids' or full-sized lifting and walking robots (Siripala 2018). The benefits of such resources, though, should be considered against the potential for misuse, intrusiveness or perhaps for them becoming a substitute for human interaction.

MOBILE APPS FOR SMARTPHONES AND TABLETS

The range of technological devices shown above is supported by the development of what are perhaps more instantly accessible resources, namely mobile apps. As with other areas of healthcare the number of available apps is increasing almost exponentially. A small selection is outlined by Young Dementia UK and are included below:

- *It's Done!* (gives reminders for daily tasks, for example, taking medication, shutting the front door or turning off the oven)
- *Jointly* (carers' app combining group messaging with to-do lists)
- *Knome* (helps to remember people's names)
- *MindMate* (designed to aid independence and quality of life)
- *Myhomehelper* (memory aid)
- *Young Onset Dementia* (gives access to appropriate information, knowledge and support).

(Young Dementia UK 2019)

Media messages

There is an abundance of media products promoting awareness and challenging attitudes concerning the experience of dementia for individuals and their families. Previous chapters featured a number of personal accounts reflecting first-hand experience. This section expands the focus, reviewing the wider range of products and narratives available across the media spectrum. It includes semi-autobiographical and fictional accounts where dementia is a central issue, motif or characteristic, which are steadily attaining greater exposure (Manthorpe 2005). What such examples offer varies according to the communicative properties of each medium and include textual, visual and auditory cues, which are subsequently accessed and decoded by interpretative recipients (Morris 2006). As can be expected, the quality and degree of accuracy and sensitivity shown by these products will be very variable. There are though some vibrant, informative and thought-provoking examples available.

Television

SOAPS

A particularly potent TV genre reaching millions of viewers on a daily basis are soap operas, or simply *the soaps*. Storylines about dementia have featured some much-loved characters who have been known to audiences for many years. This in a sense mirrors the experience of families when one of its members is diagnosed with dementia. Two relatively recent storylines in UK soaps involved Ashley (*Emmerdale*) and Mike Baldwin (*Coronation Street*).

The *Coronation Street* (2006) storyline was particularly notable in respect of the episode where Mike Baldwin received his diagnosis of dementia. The Alzheimer's Society broadcast their first TV advertisement on the day of this episode (Third Sector 2006) and subsequently received a record number of calls to their advertised helpline. Another related feature that viewers will now be very familiar with involves contact details for agencies and organizations directed 'for anyone affected by storylines in this programme', which are offered as the credits roll up the screen. This illustrates the potency of linking health promotion and advocacy initiatives with popular media products. Whilst prompting a favourable response in those seeking help, this storyline did attract some criticism. Keith Turner, *Coronation Street* fan and himself diagnosed with dementia, felt that although it was a fantastically handled storyline the speed of the character's decline was unrealistic and far too rapid (Elliot 2006). In contrast, the *Emmerdale* (2016) storyline was screened over a period of two years, providing more reality and challenging the norm for soaps where storylines commonly develop over a rapid and unrealistic timeline. This built up to a 'decisive moment' with a specially produced episode portraying scenes shot directly from Ashley's perspective. It provided an alternative reality to that of other characters who would themselves regard Ashley as acting confusedly whereas viewers offered the *point of view* shot would understand what he was relating to. It powerfully expressed Ashley's felt experience with his exasperation, bafflement, anxiety and desperation perfectly portrayed. A more conventional shooting of scenes would have perhaps focused the viewer more upon Ashley's external behaviour, which would distance them from his internal world.

DRAMA

The BBC hospital drama series *Casualty* (BBC One 2019a) has featured a storyline with one of its longest running and much-loved characters, Duffy, being diagnosed with dementia after struggling with her mood, displaying erratic behaviour and experiencing falls. Part of this show's research involved contact with Dementia UK, an approach that is being replicated more frequently by other programme makers. The consulting of individuals and groups who might be regarded as 'expert by experience' is a welcome development. Following episodes show Duffy living her life with continued productivity, offering her services as an 'expert by experience' in a care home and then as a hospital volunteer. What this storyline does well is also showcase the emotional struggle of her husband Charlie as he tries to come to terms with his own feelings. As a point of criticism, though, the rate of her subsequent decline has been perhaps too fast and could have shown more of the productive *living beyond dementia* concept.

The TV drama *Care* (BBC One 2018) featured a young single mother who is suddenly faced with her mother (Alison Steadman) having dementia following a stroke. A particular focus of this programme was the showcasing of the struggle involved for families in accessing social care support.

The 2019 TV drama *Elizabeth is Missing*, based upon Emma Healey's novel of the same name, follow's Maud's search to find out what happened to her best friend Elizabeth (BBC One 2019b). It strongly portrayed the blurring between the present and past with Maud existing within both states of time. The narrative kept us strongly within Maud's world and sphere of reference, enabling us to identify more strongly with her personal experience.

Films

Movies depicting dementia show the experience from a variety of familial perspectives and include some very highly rated films, including the Academy Award (Oscar) winning movie *A Separation* (2011). This Iranian film centred upon a married couple and their dilemma about either improving the life of their child by moving to another country or staying in Iran to look after a deteriorating parent with Alzheimer's disease.

Away from Her (2006) stars Julie Christie and Gordon Pinsent and focuses strongly upon a partner's journey after the diagnosis of dementia. In this instance, Grant's longing to connect with his wife is made all the more heart-breaking and poignant given his wife's fading cognition and later transfer of her affections to a fellow nursing home resident.

A Song for Martin (*En Sång för Martin*) (2001) is a Swedish film showcasing a couple's increasing struggle following Martin's deteriorating condition. It centres strongly upon the couple's relationship and the impact that Martin's dementia had upon both parties.

I Did Not Kill Gandhi (*Maine Gandhi Ko Nahin Mara*) (2005) is an Indian film chronicling a retired Hindi professor's experience of dementia and the impact that this has upon him and his family. The film is notable for its ending where the internal reality of the individual with dementia is acknowledged and validated through psychodramatic means.

Iris (2001) is a biopic based upon John Bayley's biographical text chronicling his wife's (Iris Murdoch) fading cognition and his own downward spiralling role as carer. It is powerfully portrayed and won an Academy Award for Jim Broadbent (playing Iris' husband).

Novels

Bernlef's (1989) *Out of Mind*, recognized as the Mind Book of the Year (1988), is a Dutch novel notable for its rich and expressive first-person narrative. The progressive change in prose style is striking, reflecting Maarten's continuing cognitive deterioration. The written narrative accordingly becomes more fragmented and less coherent yet still vividly communicating Maarten's emotional experience.

Still Alice by Lisa Genova (2007) centres around linguistics professor Alice Howland's experience of dementia. It illustrates her struggle to continue her role within the family and her occupational life. The essence of this book is in the title showing that she strives to be recognized and defined more by who she is (Alice) as opposed to her deteriorating cognitive state.

Elizabeth is Missing (2014) – Emma Healey's book (and TV drama) features Maud and her daughter Helen. Maud has dementia and is determined to uncover the mystery of her missing friend Elizabeth. This narrative highlights very powerfully the experience of shifting between different temporal states. It also highlights the family dynamic through Helen's growing concern for her mother's welfare.

Unbecoming by Jenny Downham (2016) is a novel about a family and caring. Each individual has their own dynamic they are struggling to cope with, a situation compounded by the arrival of Mary (mother and grandmother) who has dementia. A strong thread running through the book is the developing reciprocal relationship between Mary and teenage granddaughter Katie.

Jordan Elizabeth's (2016) *The Goat Children* is a tale of caring for someone with dementia. It centres eloquently around the experience of young carers following the teenage Keziah's support for her Oma (grandmother) with dementia. A notable feature is the embracing of Oma's new reality concerning the mythical goat children.

Theatre

The AZ2B Theatre Company produce and perform some wonderfully evocative plays around the experience of dementia.

Grandma, Remember Me is about three generations of a family and how they cope emotionally when one of its members has dementia.

What Do You See follows the transformation of Marshall Joan's Care Home from a failing, unhappy and stress-filled environment to one of success with a culture that cares. (https://az2btheatre.com)

STILL ALICE

This is the theatre adaptation of Lisa Genova's novel about a linguistics professor who develops dementia. It shows her moving between experiences of both struggling and coping.

DEMENTIA-FRIENDLY THEATRE PERFORMANCES

The example here is more about the environment within which plays are performed. The Leeds Playhouse, for example, regularly run dementia-friendly performances with adaptations to sound and lighting levels, extra seating, clear signage and helpers along access routes. (https://leedsplayhouse.org.uk)

Art

DEMENTIA

Karoline Hinz's 2013 (DSDC 2014) sculpture *Dementia* challenges the spectator to move beyond their preconceptions about the condition, illustrating the point that changes predominantly take place within the body and mind rather than being externally observable. It is a powerful and thought-provoking piece of art. (http://karolinehinz.com/dementia)

WILLIAM UTERMOHLEN

William Utermohlen painted a series of self-portraits from 1967, through 1996, the year of his diagnosis of Alzheimer's disease, up to 2000, charting his decline. These paintings depict a startling change of form reflecting a strong impression of his changing perceptual dynamic. (https://www.futurelearn.com/courses/dementia-arts/0/steps/44896)

MOTHER

Matthew Finn's photobook documents his mother's life over a 30-year period. It records everyday life and ordinary routines but also chronicles the onset of his mother's dementia and move from her family home into residential care. (https://mattfinn.com)

KONFETTI IM KOPF

Konfetti im Kopf (Confetti in the Head) is a national campaign in Germany raising awareness and promoting discussion around the personal experience of dementia. A core resource involves the use of photographs focusing strongly on the *person* with dementia. (https://konfetti-im-kopf.de)

Music

'I'm Not Gonna Miss You' (2014) was composed by Glen Campbell a few years following his diagnosis of Alzheimer's in 2011. This song, reflecting his own personal experience of dementia, was his last recorded song.

'Afire Love' (2014) was Ed Sheeran's tribute to his grandfather who lived with dementia for 20 years. This song reflects memories of growing up with a grandfather who lost the ability to recognize even those who were close to him. It also tenderly portrays the love between his grandparents.

'Faces of Stone' (2015) was written by Pink Floyd's David Gilmour and is about an old couple walking arm in arm. The woman suffers from memory problems and vividly recalls stories from both her youth and childhood home by the sea. She doesn't understand that she is not walking with the lover from her younger years.

Videogames

SEA HERO QUEST

Alzheimer's Research UK teamed up with Deutsche Telekom and scientists from University College London and the University of East Anglia to develop *Sea Hero Quest*, a smartphone game that rewrites the rules on how we go about dementia research. (www.alzheimersresearchuk.org/our-research/what-we-do/sea-hero-quest)

BEFORE I FORGET

In this game the player takes on the character Sunita, a woman suffering from early-onset dementia. The house is shown in monochrome with colour progressively returning as she reconnects with her past self. Examining a photograph or a piece of music provide clues to her identity. It is described in a review as: 'The video game that helped me understand my grandma's dementia' (Serrels 2018). (www.3foldgames.uk/press/before-i-forget)

Graphic Art/Cartoon Books

DAD'S NOT ALL THERE ANY MORE: A COMIC ABOUT DEMENTIA

Alex Demetris' (2016) cartoon book about his father raises awareness of dementia with Lewy bodies. Its potent learning potential is illustrated in the following review: 'I'm a doctor, and I learnt things from this comic because it is, in fact, an ideal way to learn – the reader is introduced to an individual, a family, rather than a disease or condition.'

TAKE CARE, SON: THE STORY OF MY DAD AND HIS DEMENTIA

As the title suggests, this book is about Tony Husband's father and the gradual impact that his dementia had upon him and the family (Husband 2014). Feedback for this book includes: 'Having read this book a number of times and ending up in tears, I can safely say that this is one of the most powerful books I have ever read' (Pigwig 2014).

ALICEHEIMER'S: ALZHEIMER'S THROUGH THE LOOKING GLASS

Dana Walrath's (2016) collage book about an Armenian immigrant is a *point of view* account of the experience of dementia. It has been reviewed as: 'Sometimes funny, sometimes heart-breaking'; 'illustration helps Alice's actual words subvert empathic inaccuracy, and challenge our fears' (Wojcik 2016).

How true will this be tomorrow?

The theme of 'How true will this be tomorrow?' asks you to consider current views that seek to inform the future. This commentary has an influence in informing thinking at the present time whilst also determining opinions. A number of questions will encourage you to consider its relevance, such as: have national opinions changed or not? Do you agree or not with these comments? What has influenced your attitudes?

Background information: a political and consultative vision that commenced in 2007 was published in 2009 as a National Dementia Strategy for England. This document's central tenet was to consider ways of 'living well with dementia' and offered a vision for transforming dementia services with the aim of achieving better awareness of dementia, early diagnosis and high-quality treatment at whatever stage of the illness and in whatever setting.

- A decade since this political vision, do you feel present-day dementia care services in England have improved at local and national levels?
- What evidence have you to support your responses?
- What is your understanding of the present national dementia strategies for Scotland, Wales and Northern Ireland? What are their future strategies?
- What evidence have you to support your responses?
- Who do you feel are the dementia champion experts and why?

Concluding thoughts

In this chapter we have moved beyond the Lawrence family's experience, taking a look at some of the many inspiring initiatives and campaigns championing dementia. These include some timely and much-needed approaches that are intended to accompany and brighten the journey embarked on by those with dementia and their families. The *champions* covered within this chapter and elsewhere in this text include individuals, groups, initiatives, campaigns, resources and products. The value of these cannot be underestimated or understated as they offer perhaps what could be considered as potentially the most important commodity, that of hope. This championing of dementia began with the work of notable individuals including Tom Kitwood (personhood) and Naomi Feil (validation). These ground-breaking initiatives laid the foundations for subsequent projects, as detailed throughout this chapter, which aim to reduce stigma and raise awareness around the lived experience of dementia. The number of such examples is developing at a steady rate with some truly inspiring approaches noted. This includes the addition of some thought-provoking and impactful fictional products. It is to be hoped that such initiatives as those featured above will continue to be created, expanding our understanding and focus upon the people living with dementia in their midst.

This is the final time you are asked to itemize your personal learning on the ways you, your health and social care community and the country you live in have moved towards a new age of dementia care, albeit as the decades-old words of pioneers such as Tom Kitwood and the Bradford Dementia Group continue to resonate in our present thoughts.

PERSONAL LEARNING

What was your past knowledge and understanding, what new learning have you achieved and how could this inform your future personal and/or professional interventions?

As a person involved in dementia care, my new learning includes

....

On reading the first-person narratives, my new learning includes

....

INTERVENTIONS

Be mindful that whatever comments are offered should be realistic, achievable and person-centred. Also, that the feelings conveyed and observations made reinforce the 'optimism of championing dementia care' for the individual and significant other people in their life.

Consider the types of physical intervention that could promote this

....

Consider the types of social interventions that could promote this

....

Consider the types of psychological interventions that could promote this...

....

Based on your responses, how would you know how successful you are?

....

....

References

Alzheimer's Disease International (2016). *Dementia Friendly Communities: Key Principles.* Accessed on 7/5/17 at www.alz.co.uk/adi/pdf/dfc-principles.pdf.

Alzheimer's Research (n.d.). *Play Sea Hero Quest and #gameforgood.* Accessed on 3/12/19 at www.alzheimersresearchuk.org/our-research/what-we-do/sea-hero-quest.

Alzheimer's Society (2008). *Dementia: Out of the Shadows.* Accessed on 7/5/17 at www.alzheimers.org.uk/sites/default/files/2018-08/out_of_the_shadows.pdf?fileID=454.

Alzheimer's Society (2017). Dementia Friendly Screenings: a Guide for Cinemas. Accessed 19/6/22 at https://www.alzheimers.org.uk/sites/default/files/2018-04/DFS_Guide_for_cinemas_13_TEXT_ONLY_FINAL_29NOV_1515.pdf.

Alzheimer's Society (2020). 'Side by Side.' Accessed on 15/7/20 at https://www.alzheimers.org.uk/get-support/your-support-services/side-by-side.

Alzheimer's Society Memory Walk (2020). 'Be Part of Memory Walk.' Accessed on 15/7/20 at https://www.memorywalk.org.uk.

Alzheimer's Society (2019a). *Telling the Truth to People with Dementia.* Accessed on 17/11/19 at www.alzheimers.org.uk/get-support/daily-living/making-decisions-telling-truth.

Alzheimer's Society. (2019b). *Assistive Technology and Dementia.* Accessed on 5/10/19 at www.alzheimers.org.uk/get-support/staying-independent/assistive-technology-and-dementia.

August, Bille (dir.) (2001). *A Song for Martin* [Film]. Sweden: RKO Helkon Media.

Barua, Jahnu (dir.) (2005). *I Did Not Kill Gandhi* [Film]. India: Curtain Call Co.

BAT (n.d.). *Bounce for Alzheimer's.* Accessed on 15/9/18 at www.batfoundation.com.

Batson, P., Thorne, K. and Peak, J. (2002). 'Life story work sees the person beyond the dementia.' *Journal of Dementia Care 10* (3), 15–7.

BBC One (2009). *Can Gerry Robinson Fix Dementia Care Homes?* 8 December.

BBC One (2018). *Care.* 9 December.

BBC One (2019a). *Casualty.* 7 December.

BBC One (2019b). *Elizabeth is Missing.* 8 December.

Bernlef, J. (1989). *Out of Mind.* London: Faber and Faber.

Brooker, D. (2003). 'What is person-centred care in dementia?' *Reviews in Clinical Gerontology 13*, 215–222.

Bryden, C. (2005). *Dancing with Dementia.* London: Jessica Kingsley Publishers.

Bryden, C. (2018). *Will I Still Be Me? Finding a Continuing Sense of Self in the Lived Experience of Dementia.* London: Jessica Kingsley Publishers.

Bugental, J. (1963). 'Humanistic psychology – a new breakthrough.' *American Psychologist 18* (9), 563–567.

Butler, R. (1963). 'The life review: an interpretation of reminiscence in the aged.' *Psychiatry 26* (1), 65–76.

Butterfly Household Model (n.d.). *Butterfly Household Model.* Accessed on 19/9/19 at www.dementiacarematters.com.

Campbell, G. (2014). 'I'm Not Gonna Miss You' [Sound recording]. USA: Big Machine Label Group.

Channel 4 (2015). *Dementiaville.* 28 May.

Chiang, K., Chu, H., Chang, H., Chung, M., Chen, C., Chiou, H. and Chou, K. (2010). 'The effects of reminiscence therapy on psychological well-being, depression, and loneliness among the institutionalized aged.' *International Journal of Geriatric Psychiatry 25* (4), 380–388.

Clarke, A. Hanson, E. and Ross, H. (2003). 'Seeing the person behind the patient: enhancing the care of older people using a biographical approach.' *Journal of Clinical Nursing, 12*, 697–706.

Clarke, P., Mapes, N., Burt, J. and Preston, S. (2013). 'Greening Dementia – a literature review of the benefits and barriers facing individuals living with dementia in accessing the natural environment and local greenspace.' *Natural England Commissioned Reports, 137*, 5.

Clasper, K. (2014). *Dementia Friendly Transport.* Accessed on 12/4/19 at http://ken-kenc2.blogspot.com/2014.

Clasper, K. (2017). *Dementia Friendly Banks.* Accessed on 12/4/19 at https://ken-kenc2.blogspot.com/2017/12/dementia-friendly-banks.html.

Crampton, J., Dean, J. and Eley, R. (2012). *Creating a Dementia Friendly York: Joseph Rowntree Foundation.* Accessed on 16/3/19 at www.jrf.org.uk/report/creating-dementia-friendly-york.

Dementia Care Matters (n.d.). *Dementia Care Matters.* Accessed on 6/5/19 at www.dementiacarematters.com.

Demetris, A. (2016). *Dad's Not All There Any More: A Comic About Dementia.* London: Jessica Kingsley Publishers.

Department of Health and Social Care (2009). *Living Well with Dementia: A National Dementia Strategy.* London: Department of Health and Social Care.

Downham, J. (2016). *Unbecoming.* Oxford: David Fickling Books.

Doyle, P. and Rubenstein, R. (2014). 'Person-centred dementia care and the cultural matrix of othering.' *The Gerontologist 54* (6), 952–963.

DSDC (2014). *Sculpting the Intangible: Karoline Hinz's Dementia.* Accessed on 15/12/19 at www.dementia.stir.ac.uk/blogs/diametric/2014-11-24/sculpting-intangible-karoline-hinzs-dementia.

Elizabeth, J. (2016). *The Goat Children.* USA: CHBB Publishing.

Elliot, J. (2006). 'Mike Baldwin told my dementia story.' Accessed on 14/6/2010 at news.bbc.co.uk/1/hi/health/4882156.stm.

Eyre, Richard (dir.) (2001). *Iris* [Film]. UK: Fox Iris Productions.

Farhadi, Asghar (dir.) (2011). *A Separation* [Film]. Iran: Asghar Farhadi Productions.

Fazio, S., Pace, D., Flinner, J. and Kallymer, B. (2018). 'The fundamentals of person-centered care for individuals with dementia.' *The Gerontologist, 58* (Issue supplement 1), S10–S19.

Feil, N. (2013). *The Validation Breakthrough: Simple Techniques for Communicating with People with Alzheimer's-type Dementia (3rd edition).* London: Health Professions Press.

Feil, N. (2014). 'Validation Therapy with late-onset dementia populations.' In G. Jones and B. Miesen (eds) *Care Giving in Dementia.* London: Routledge.

Fernandes, E. (2012). *Dementiaville: how an experimental new town is taking the elderly back to their happier and healthier pasts with astonishing results.* Accessed on 6/1/20 at www.dailymail.co.uk/news/article-2109801/Dementiaville-How-experimental-new-town-taking-elderly-happier-healthier-pasts-astonishing-results.html.

Future Learn (n.d.). 'William Utermohlen and his self-portraits.' Accessed on 15/7/20 at https://www.futurelearn.com/courses/dementia-arts/0/steps/44896.

Genova, L. (2007). *Still Alice.* London: Simon and Schuster.

Gibson, F. (2004). *The Past in the Present: Using Reminiscence in Health and Social Care.* Baltimore: Health Professions Press.

Gilmour, D. (2015). 'Faces of Stone.' [Sound recording]. UK: Columbia.

Guardian, The (2015). 'Christopher Eccleston: "Dementia dismantled my father's personality."' 31 May. Accessed on 17/3/17 at www.theguardian.com/lifeandstyle/2015/may/31/christopher-eccleston-father-dementia-disease-dismantled-his-personality.

Healey, E. (2014). *Elizabeth is Missing.* London: Penguin.

Heathcote, J. (2009). 'Memories are made of this: reminiscence activities for person-centred care.' London: Alzheimer's Society.

Hinz, K. (2013). *Dementia.* [Plaster and amethyst sculpture]. Accessed on 19/6/20 at http://karolinehinz.com/dementia.

Husband, T. (2014). *Take Care, Son: The Story of My Dad and His Dementia.* London: Constable and Robinson.

Innovations in Dementia (n.d.). *Innovations in Dementia.* Accessed on 6/3/19 at www.innovationsindementia.org.uk.

ITV1 (2006). *Coronation Street.* 7 April.

ITV1 (2016). *Emmerdale.* 20 December.

Jackson, D. (2010). 'The most difficult decision in my life.' In L. Whitman (ed.) *Telling Tales About Dementia: Experiences of Caring.* London: Jessica Kingsley Publishers.

Jeraj, S. and Butt, J. (2018). *Dementia and Black, Asian and Minority Ethnic Communities.* Accessed on 6/10/19 at www.dementiaaction.org.uk/assets/0004/0379/Dementia_and_BAME_Communities_report_Final_v2.pdf.

Kitwood, T. (1988). 'The technical, the personal, and the framing of dementia.' *Social Behaviour 3,* 161–179.

Kitwood, T. (1997). *Dementia Reconsidered: The Person Comes First.* Buckingham: Open University Press.

Kitwood, T. (1998). 'Toward a theory of dementia care: ethics and interaction.' *The Journal of Clinical Ethics 9,* 23–34.

Kitwood, T. and Bredin, K. (1992). 'Towards a theory of dementia care: personhood and well-being.' *Ageing and Society 12,* 269–287.

Kogan, A.C., Wilber, K. and Mosquedo, L. (2016). 'Person-centered care for older adults with chronic conditions and functional impairment: a systematic literature review.' *Journal of the American Geriatrics Society 64,* 1–7.

Leeds Playhouse (2018). Dementia Friendly Performance. Accessed on 12/7/19 at https://leedsplayhouse.org.uk/wp-content/uploads/2018/11/Dementia-Friendly-leaflet-online-version.pdf?dm_i=2YIG,SM9U,5SBZFW,2Y5HR,1.

Manthorpe, J. (2005). 'A child's eye view: dementia in children's literature.' *British Journal of Social Work 35* (3), 305–320.

Mapes, N., Milton, S., Nicholls, V. and Williamson, T. (2016). *Is It Nice Outside? Consulting People Living with Dementia and Carers About Engaging with the Natural Environment.* Natural England Commissioned Reports, Number 211.

Maslow, A. (1943). 'A theory of human motivation.' *Psychological Review 50* (1), 370–396.

Maslow, A. (1970). *Motivation and Personality (2nd edition).* New York: Evanston.

McKee, K., Wilson, F., Elford, H., Hinchliff, S., Bolton, G., Chung, M. and Goudie, F. (2003). 'Reminiscence: is living in the past good for wellbeing?' *Nursing and Residential Care 5,* 489–491.

McKeown, J., Clarke, A. and Repper, J. (2006). 'Life story work in health and social care: systematic literature review.' *Journal of Advanced Nursing 55,* 237–247.

McNair, D., Cunningham, C. and Pollock, R. (2010). *Light and Lighting Design for People with Dementia.* Stirling: Dementia Services Development Centre.

Memory Box Network (n.d.). *Memory Box Network*. Accessed on 12/3/19 at www.memoryboxnetwork.org.

Memory Walk (n.d.). *Memory Walk*. Accessed on 15/6/19 at www.alzheimers.org.uk.

Moos, I. and Bjorn, A. (2006). 'Use of life story in the institutional care of people with dementia: a review of intervention studies.' *Ageing and Society 26*, 431–454.

Morris, G. (2006). *Mental Health Issues and the Media*. London: Routledge.

Morris, G. and Morris, J. (2010). *The Dementia Care Workbook*. Berkshire: Open University Press.

Murphy, C. (2000). *Crackin' lives: an evaluation of a life story book project to assist patients from a long stay psychiatric hospital in their move to community care situations*. Stirling: Dementia Services Development Centre.

Noack, R. (2017). 'A German nursing home tries a novel form of dementia therapy: Re-creating a vanished era for its patients.' 26 December. Accessed on 6/11/19 at www.washingtonpost.com/news/worldviews/wp/2017/12/26/a-german-nursing-home-tries-a-novel-form-of-dementia-therapy-re-creating-a-vanished-era-for-its-patients/?noredirect=on&utm_term=.48c70d1c6c52.

Oxford English Dictionary (2020). Accessed on 6/1/20 at www.oed.com.

Pietrukowicz, M. and Johnson, M. (1991). 'Using life histories to individualise nursing home staff attitudes towards residents.' *The Gerontologist 31*, 105–6.

Pigwig (2014). *Review of Husband Take Care, Son: The Story of My Dad and His Dementia*. Accessed on 12/9/19 at www.amazon.co.uk.

Polley, Sarah (dir.) (2006). *Away from Her* [Film]. USA: Foundry Pictures.

Pollock, A. (2014a). 'Meaningful outdoor spaces for people with dementia.' In E. Feddersen and I. Lüdtke (eds) *Lost in Space: Architecture in Dementia*. Basel: Birkhäuser.

Pollock, R. (2014b). 'Architectural Space, Acoustics and Dementia.' In E. Feddersen and I. Lüdtke (eds) *Lost in Space: Architecture in Dementia*. Basel: Birkhäuser.

Reagan, R. (1994). *Text of letter written by President Ronald Reagan announcing he has Alzheimer's disease*. Accessed on 6/8/18 at www.reaganlibrary.gov/sreference/reagan-s-letter-announcing-his-alzheimer-s-diagnosis.

RIBA (2017). *Designing for Specialist Dementia Care*. Accessed on 5/2/19 at www.architecture.com/knowledge-and-resources/knowledge-landing-page/designing-for-specialist-dementia-care.

Rogers, C. (1946). 'Significant aspects of client-centred therapy.' *American Psychologist 1*, 415–422.

Rogers, C. (1961). *On Becoming a Person*. London: Constable and Robinson.

Rogers, C. (1967). *On Becoming a Person: A Therapist's View of Psychotherapy*. London: Constable.

Schofield, I. and Tolson, D. (2010). *Scottish Football Museum Reminiscence Pilot Project for People with Dementia*. Glasgow: Glasgow Caledonian University.

Schweitzer, P. and Bruce, E. (2008). *Remembering Yesterday, Caring Today: Reminiscence in Dementia Care, a Guide to Good Practice*. London: Jessica Kingsley Publishers.

Serrels, M. (2018). *The video game that helped me understand my grandma's dementia*. Accessed on 18/1/19 at www.cnet.com/news/the-video-game-that-helped-me-understand-my-grandmas-dementia.

Sheeran, E. (2014). 'Afire Love.' [Sound recording]. UK: Asylum.

Siripala, T. (2018). 'Japan's robot revolution in senior care.' 9 June. Accessed on at www.japantimes.co.jp/opinion/2018/06/09/commentary/japan-commentary/japans-robot-revolution-senior-care/#.XepoyZP7SM8.

Spector, A., Orrell, M., Davies, S. and Woods, R. (2004). 'Reminiscence therapy for dementia.' *The Cochrane Database of Systematic Reviews 1*, 1–14.

Sporting Memories (n.d.). *Sporting Memories*. Accessed on 8/2/19 at www.sportingmemoriesnetwork.com/news/pfa-practical-guide-to-living-with-dementia.

Telegraph, The (2008). 'Fake bus stop keeps Alzheimer's patients from wandering off.' 3 June. Accessed on 8/4/19 at www.telegraph.co.uk/news/newstopics/howaboutthat/2071319/Fake-bus-stop-keeps-Alzheimers-patients-from-wandering-off.html.

Telegraph, The (2015). 'Is letting dementia patients live in the past the best form of care?' 4 June. Accessed on 16/5/17 at www.telegraph.co.uk/news/health/elder/11649751/Is-letting-dementia-patients-live-in-the-past-the-best-form-of-care.html.

Third Sector (2006). *Third Sector*. Accessed on 8/10/18 at www.thirdsector.co.uk.

Turpie, S. (2017). 'Dementia Friendly Housing: an architect's perspective.' Accessed on 16/3/19 at dementia.stir.ac.uk/blogs/dementia-centred/2017-11-08/dementia-friendly-housing-architects-perspective.

Walrath, D. (2016). *Aliceheimer's: Alzheimer's Through the Looking Glass (Graphic Medicine)*. Pennsylvania: Pennsylvania State University Press.

Weller, C. (2017). 'Inside the Dutch "dementia village" that offers beer, bingo and top notch healthcare.' Accessed on 6/10/18 at www.uk.businessinsider.com/inside-hogewey-dementia-village-2017-7/#staff-at-hogeweyk-are-trained-to-focus-on-highlighting-what-residents-can-do-not-what-they-cant-2.

Wojcik, E. (2016). *Massachusetts Review*. Accessed on 6/7/19 at www.massreview.org/node/581.

Woods, R., Bruce, E., Edwards, R., Elvish, R., Hoare, Z., Hounsome, B., Keady, J., Moniz-Cook, E., Orgeta, V., Orrell, M., Rees, J. and Russell, I. (2012). 'REMCARE: reminiscence groups for people with dementia and their family caregivers – effectiveness and cost-effectiveness pragmatic multicentre randomised trial.' *Health Technology Assessment 16* (48), 1–116.

Woods, R., Bruce, E., Edwards, R., Hounsome, B., Keady, J., Moniz-Cook, E., Orrell, M. and Russell, I. (2009). 'Reminiscence groups for people with dementia and their family carers: pragmatic eight-centre randomised trial of joint reminiscence and maintenance versus usual treatment: a protocol.' *Trials 30* (10), 64.

Woods, R., Portnoy, S., Head, D. and Jones, G. (1992). *Care Giving in Dementia: Research and Applications*. London: Routledge.

Young Dementia UK (2019). *Helpful Technology*. Accessed on 18/6/19 at www.youngdementiauk.org/helpful-technology.

Chapter 8

Exercises

More than a decade ago, we began collecting feedback from healthcare students prior to, during and on completion of their clinical placements in dementia care settings. This involved visiting people in the community, day care and residential care. We were also involved in the monitoring and auditing of local mental health services for people with dementia.

Figure 8.1 identifies a series of concerns from that time and we include them for the reader to reflect on their present practice and observations from contact with dementia services.

Low staff morale

Time restrictions influencing practice

Lack of resources (human, financial, attitudes)

Care teams sometimes mismanaged

Students' ideals re: person-centred approaches and actual practice often differed

Negative attitudes towards dementia care services

Figure 8.1 Practice concerns

Your reflections concerning Figure 8.1 could be enhanced by considering the following questions:

- What are your views on these earlier comments?
- Do you feel some or all of these comments are still valid today?
- If so, which cause you the most concern?
- If they are no longer valid, what approaches need to be maintained to prevent their reappearance?

Reflection should be about thinking and learning from experiences and making use of the learning in the future. Boud and Walker (1998) have argued that reflection should enable learners to express doubts, uncertainty and awareness of contradictions. The 'publishing' of interpretations within small groups encourages personal declarations and attending to colleagues' thoughts, feelings and beliefs.

Each of the preceding seven chapters has encouraged the reader to explore and express their personal reflections through structured questions and activities. This promoted assessment of knowledge, understanding and ways of engagement concerning the reader:

- in a number of familial roles as a member of the Lawrence family
- as an observer of other people's felt experiences
- in their consideration of interventions that could be employed (realistic, achievable and person-centred approaches).

This three-stage reflective approach is based on what the reader has already considered or documented, namely what their past knowledge, understanding and attitudes were, and what new learning they have achieved. Schön (1991) argued that professionals in their everyday practice face unique and complex situations that are unsolvable by adopting technical rational approaches alone, proposing an approach where professionals' learning is facilitated by reflection. This process assists in providing insightful learning opportunities by the use of structured activities that allow healthcare students to reflect on their own attitudes and listen to interpretations from peers.

In Chapter 3 we briefly asked you for your values, beliefs and attitudes to the series of questions shown in Figure 8.2.

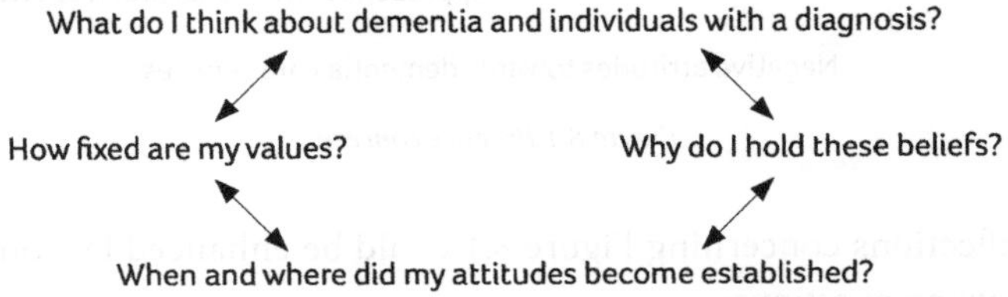
What do I think about dementia and individuals with a diagnosis?
How fixed are my values?
Why do I hold these beliefs?
When and where did my attitudes become established?

Figure 8.2 Personal beliefs

We would like you to now revisit and reflect further upon your initial responses. Below are a number of factors that could influence your past, present or future thoughts:

- Did your age and life experiences influence your response?
- Is familial knowledge or personal awareness significant regarding your responses?
- What professional knowledge is required for you to better understand dementia?

The art of reflection can often be enhanced by having the opportunity to listen to others' interpretations. You may have limited experience or regular opportunities to learn in group settings where there is a sharing of education and discussions, rather than more didactic/passive forms of learning. We are mindful that this educational style may not suit every reader or be a learning approach that is accessible. However, we include some thoughts and structures relating to ways of working in shared learning groups.

When considering the ways of working or facilitating structured exercises within learning groups certain boundaries should be first explored with the participants. Each person is asked to contribute in devising some ground rules that influence or determine the conduct of participants by seeking responses to what are *acceptable* and *unacceptable* behaviours. Examples could include the following.

Acceptable behaviours:

- maintaining confidentiality
- showing respect
- listening to each other
- being non-judgemental
- offering constructive feedback
- being punctual.

Unacceptable behaviours:

- talking over each other
- showing intolerance towards each other
- ignoring each other
- poor time keeping
- rude behaviours.

These ground rules around *acceptable* and *unacceptable* behaviours provide participants with the types of behaviours that either promote or inhibit contributions. Discussions and clarifications can be explored around a number of important themes, for example maintaining boundaries of confidentiality.

The model of experiential learning developed by Kolb (1984) suggests that the process of learning consists of four phases. We have adapted and modified the experiential learning approach in order to allow healthcare students the opportunity to explore their values and attitudes towards people with dementia:

- *concrete experience* (occurs when the person is involved in carrying out a task)
- *reflection* (a personal reflection on that experience)
- *abstract conceptualization* (a process that involves identifying general rules describing the experience, or the application of known theories to it, which leads to ideas about ways of modifying the next occurrence of the experience)
- *active experimentation* (represents the application of these new skills or ideas in practice, which in turn leads to a new set of concrete experiences, which are in turn reflected on).

In essence when a person carries out some type of action they have an opportunity to observe and reflect upon its underlying processes and consider the possible consequences. Subsequently, this action can become open to the person theorizing and forming some general outcomes. This can then be further tested through new experiences in order to both validate their actions and develop them further. Self-awareness allows a person to analyse their feelings honestly and to examine how the situation has affected the individual, and how the individual has affected the situation (Schön 1991).

The exercises in this chapter have been designed in an informal and constructive manner so that the reader can appreciate structure and process. Furthermore this formula can be transferred in order to facilitate opportunities in student-centred learning. After every exercise we include a brief series of headings for the teacher/facilitator(s) to reflect upon the learning process.

EXERCISE: HEALTH CONCERNS (CHAPTER 1)

AIM

This exercise encourages health and social care professionals (qualified or student) to explore their understanding of what could necessitate a 'health concern' from an eclectic approach.

RESOURCES

- worksheets
- three sheets of poster paper, pens, pins/paper adhesive
- cue cards
- an environment free from distractions (for example, clutter, noise) with an ambient temperature and appropriate seating.

STRUCTURES

Provide worksheets to the participants asking them to decide their understanding of their own eclectic approach under three headings: Physical, Psychological, Social.

For example, physical factors (disease, trauma, genetic), psychological factors (mental health, well-being), social factors (environmental, familial, financial). Participants are then encouraged to write their comments on poster paper under the three respective headings.

Collective interpretations are then placed in full view for discussion.

In pairs, participants identify a 'health concern', giving time for discussion as to why this could be an issue. Being mindful of the agreed ways of working (e.g. confidentiality), ask participants a concern that can relate to themselves or a friend.

Provide participants with worksheets so that they can write down the impact the identified 'health concern' could have in both an internal (self) and external (other people and that person's environment) lifestyle.

Health concern	
Impact on self	Impact on others

Following this paired activity encourage group feedback and then allow time for discussions to be written up on the respective poster papers. Having generated a range of personal eclectic approaches, introduce structured 'health concerns' in the form of cue cards, for example, memory problems or disinhibited behaviours, that can be distributed to participants in either similar or different small groups.

Provide time for discussion using the comments already written on the poster papers as a structure for exploring how a 'health concern' can have an impact on the person especially when they feel that 'something is wrong'.

VARIATIONS

Ask participants to provide examples from their clinical/social practice settings (maintaining confidentiality) on a person's health concerns.

TEACHER/FACILITATOR(S) REFLECTIONS

- group's ways of working
- beginnings
- process observations
- closing
- overall evaluation(s).

EXERCISE: ON BEING TESTED (CHAPTER 2)

AIM

This exercise encourages health and social care professionals (qualified or student) to explore their understanding of the 'felt experiences of being tested'.

RESOURCES

- worksheets
- poster paper, pens, pins/paper adhesive
- cue cards
- an environment free from distractions (for example, clutter, noise) with an ambient temperature and appropriate seating.

STRUCTURES

In pairs, give participants worksheets and ask them to reflect on times when they were involved in being tested (e.g. medical examinations, driving lessons, academic examinations). This is aimed at generating a joint list of these tests and a highlighting of their feelings before and after a 'test'.

Types of test(s)

Feelings before...

Feelings afterwards...

Lasting thoughts...

In groups, participants are encouraged to provide a list on poster paper of the range of tests discussed (but avoiding their feelings and lasting thoughts). Write down on each cue card one of these tests. Ask participants to get into small groups allocating Participant A as *being tested*, Participant B as *the tester* and other participants as observers. It might be helpful to ask the observers to briefly decide what they could observe, for example, how the testing process commenced; how it was managed (whether prompts/encouragement were used); how closure was conducted. Observations are written down on a worksheet.

Allow enough time for participants to experience each of the three roles and provide feedback (that is e.g. constructive, realistic and achievable).

Encourage general discussions on these three opportunities for involvement in the testing process, and the range of feelings each of these roles generated for the participants.

Ask participants to look back on their original worksheets and compare comments with those made when being an observer.

General discussions on the participants' comments can be facilitated acknowledging which approaches could be used to lessen negative feelings and promote positive ones.

VARIATIONS

Provide examples from clinical/social practice care (maintaining confidentiality) on the approaches used to test and assess a person, for example, memory, concentration, cognitive function.

TEACHER/FACILITATOR(S) REFLECTIONS

- group's ways of working
- beginnings
- process observations
- closing
- overall evaluation(s).

EXERCISE: WHAT IF IT'S NOT ALZHEIMER'S DISEASE? (CHAPTER 3)

AIM

This exercise encourages health and social care professionals (qualified or student) to explore their 'felt experiences' and understanding of the ways vascular dementia is researched, causative lifestyles and narratives.

RESOURCES

- worksheets
- access and time to use the internet
- poster paper, pens, pins/paper adhesive
- an environment free from distractions (for example, clutter, noise) with an ambient temperature and appropriate seating.

STRUCTURES

Convene a brief discussion on what is collectively known about vascular dementia in order to discover the participants' knowledge and/or practical experiences. A worksheet is provided for each person with a series of questions.

Ask the group to form three small groups. Allocate a theme to each group and agree how long an internet search would take. If this facility is unavailable we suggest time in a library.

What is vascular dementia?

- causative factors and unhealthy lifestyles
- research and funding arrangements (local/national)
- narratives on the lived experiences e.g. blogs.

On reconvening, allow time for small group feedback and discussions on how easy or difficult it was to collect information. What new knowledge was discovered? Where does funding come from and how is it distributed? How insightful were the first-person narratives?

As part of an extended learning project you could encourage the compiling of a local resource. Again in small groups, depending on size and time, encourage the collection of information on self-help organizations, social and charitable events, local media reporting, and the ways hospitals and surgeries provide information on dementia. On reconvening, allow time for small group feedback and the collective production of a resource pack of local facilities.

VARIATIONS

Depending on the group's awareness and understanding of vascular dementia you could consider other types of dementia, for example, Korsakoff's syndrome, fronto-temporal dementia or dementia with Lewy bodies.

TEACHER/FACILITATOR(S) REFLECTIONS

- group's ways of working
- beginnings
- process observations
- closing
- overall evaluation(s).

EXERCISE: CHANGING RELATIONSHIPS ON BECOMING A CARER (CHAPTER 4)

AIM

This exercise encourages health and social care professionals (qualified or student) to explore their understanding of the ways relationships can change when becoming a carer.

RESOURCES

- cue cards
- worksheets
- poster paper, pens, pins/paper adhesive
- an environment free from distractions (for example, clutter, noise) with an ambient temperature and appropriate seating.

STRUCTURES

Depending on the size of the group, ask participants to organize themselves in smaller groups of two, three or four. Distribute half of these groups a cue card saying:

> What do you think it could mean to become a carer?

Then distribute to the other groups a different cue card saying:

> What could 'get in the way' if you became a carer?

If the setting is conducive, separate the sets of groups so that they cannot hear the ensuing discussions, or ask their contributions to be said quietly. Allocate time so that each person has an opportunity to reply to the cue card question. One person takes the responsibility of writing the responses. In turn ask each group to present their findings and allow time for general discussion.

Now distribute a worksheet to each group with the following question:

> **If I became a family/partner carer, how could this influence my:**
>
> – new relationships?
> – new roles?
> – intimacy?

1. Decide the family status of the person diagnosed i.e. mum or dad, and your status i.e. son or daughter.
2. If the small groups would prefer, explore the possible dynamics between partners.

In turn ask each group to present their findings and allow time for general discussion.

VARIATIONS

We do not wish to be prescriptive but allowing the participants access to published material could substantiate their findings/discussions. You may wish to direct the reading matter but here are some pertinent examples of carers:

- Carling, C. (2012). *But Then Something Happened*. Cambridge: Golden Books.
- Suchet, J. (2010). *My Bonnie*. London: Harper.

TEACHER/FACILITATOR(S) REFLECTIONS

- group's ways of working
- beginnings
- process observations
- closing
- overall evaluation(s).

EXERCISE: CRISIS AND THE YOUNG CARER (CHAPTER 5)

AIM

This exercise encourages health and social care professionals (qualified or student) to explore their personal thoughts, feelings and possible behaviours about being a 'young carer'. By exploring these personal dynamics, regardless of your own age, you are asked to contemplate a 'life crisis' and how this could influence your interpretations.

RESOURCES

- worksheets
- poster paper, pens, pins/paper adhesive
- an environment free from distractions (for example, clutter, noise) with an ambient temperature and appropriate seating.

STRUCTURES

Distribute Worksheet 1 to each person in the group.

Worksheet 1
Identify a life experience that has caused you to have feelings of being in crisis. At that time, what were your:

- thoughts?
- feelings?
- behaviours?

Knowledge of the participants and how the group functions, for example ground rules, is an important consideration. If appropriate, ask for small groups (twos or threes) and decide what information they would be willing to share. Allow time for feedback and then general discussion. If not suitable, provide the group with a 'life crisis' and have a general discussion on thoughts, feelings and behaviours.

Distribute Worksheet 2 to each person in the group.

Worksheet 2
Personal information

- Where did you live?
- Who did you live with?
- How did you spend your time?
- What were your interests?

Ask participants to consider their present age and if relevant deduct 10 or 20 years or more. Now reflect on when you were a young person (teenager). Ask participants to form small groups but make them now, where possible, age specific.

Being mindful of what has been mentioned above regarding ways of working, ask participants to consider what information they are willing to share and encourage discussion. Then ask these small groups to discuss what thoughts, feelings and behaviours could result if they were a young carer. Convene a general discussion around the topic of 'What approaches could be employed towards the adult person who has a diagnosis of dementia?'

VARIATIONS

We do not wish to be prescriptive but allowing the participants access to published material could substantiate their findings/ discussions. You may wish to direct the reading matter. We include two pertinent examples you could use:

- A teenager speaks out about the strain of being a young carer (Alzheimer's Society 2016).
- Young People Caring for Adults with Dementia in England: Report on NCB's Survey Findings and Internet Research (National Children's Bureau 2016).

TEACHER/FACILITATOR(S) REFLECTIONS

- group's ways of working
- beginnings
- process observations
- closing
- overall evaluation(s).

EXERCISE: IN SEARCH OF 'DEMENTIA FRIENDLINESS' (CHAPTER 6)

AIM

An exercise in two or more parts, it encourages health and social care professionals (qualified or student) to reflect and debate the theme 'dementia friendly'. Exploration of community provisions would require contact with local health and social care services and if appropriate access to the internet.

RESOURCES

- worksheets
- poster paper, pens, pins/paper adhesive
- an environment free from distractions (for example, clutter, noise) with an ambient temperature and appropriate seating.

STRUCTURES

At the initial meeting provide each participant with a worksheet. After completion encourage a general discussion. If relevant, provide the views of successive government policies, for example, the first National Dementia Strategy *Living Well with Dementia* (Department of Health and Social Care 2009) or *The Prime Minister's Challenge on Dementia 2020* (Department of Health 2015).

'Dementia friendly'

- What is your understanding?
- When did you first hear this term?
- Has it a presence in your community?
- Which organizations promote this approach?

Document the participants' comments on poster paper for referral at a later time. Organize into, ideally, four small groups, with specific remits around promoting 'dementia-friendly' approaches including what, where, when and how these initiatives were established, for example, separate group(s) discovering health and/or social care services, charities and local organizations. Provide appropriate time for participants to discover these social facilities in their community.

Health, social, charity or local organizations

- What are these initiatives?
- Where can they be found?
- When were they established?
- How are they organized?

The second meeting will establish the findings from the small groups. Ask each group to nominate a spokesperson and rearrange the furniture into a 'discussion forum' with the remaining participants becoming the audience.

Ask each nominee to present their findings with the audience being supportive of their comments. These discussions should also allow for what was encouraging and/or disappointing about discovering these local facilities. On completion of all the presentations ask the participants to revisit their original comments on 'dementia friendly' and open up for general discussions to see if individual interpretations and earlier documentation on poster paper complemented the group findings or not.

VARIATIONS

Based upon the participants findings, asks them to consider:

- What is realistic and can be achieved by 2020?
- What appears to be unrealistic by 2020?

TEACHER/FACILITATOR(S) REFLECTIONS

- group's ways of working
- beginnings
- process observations
- closing
- overall evaluation(s).

References

Alzheimer's Society (2016). 'A teenager speaks out about the strain of being a young carer.' Accessed on 15/7/20 at https://www.alzheimers.org.uk/get-support/publications-and-factsheets/dementia-together-magazine/young-carer.

Boud, D. and Walker, D. (1998). 'Promoting reflection in professional courses: the challenge of context.' *Studies in Higher Education 23* (2), 191–206.

Carling, C. (2012). *But Then Something Happened*. Cambridge: Golden Books.

Department of Health (2015). *The Prime Minister's Challenge on Dementia 2020*. London: DHSC.

Department of Health and Social Care (2009). *Living Well with Dementia*. London: Department of Health and Social Care.

Kolb, D.A. (1984). *Experiential Learning Experience as the Source of Learning and Development*. Englewood Cliffs, NJ: Prentice-Hall.

Morris, G. and Morris, J. (2010). *The Dementia Care Workbook*. Berkshire: Open University Press.

National Children's Bureau (2016). *Young People Caring for Adults with Dementia in England: Report on NCB's Survey Findings and Internet Research*. London: National Children's Bureau.

Schön, D. (1991). *The Reflective Practitioner (2nd edition)*. San Francisco: Jossey Bass.

Suchet, J. (2010). *My Bonnie*. London: Harper.

Concluding Thoughts

This book emerged out of conversations between the authors that have taken place over many years and that ultimately engage you, the reader. Our initial dialogue shaped the early directions of the themes relating to relationships and dementia, but always wanting to remind the reader of the uniqueness of the person when in receipt of this all-encompassing diagnosis. However, if that person is in a relationship then significant others will be touched by the diagnosis and remain a witness to change. This led to the focus of this work extending to and embracing the whole family, recognizing that each member had their own personal experience and that in a number of cases support needs remain unmet. It acknowledges the concept of a dementia diagnosis being received by the whole family unit as opposed to just the person with dementia or the person with dementia and their partner. The authors have for a long time been concerned about those individuals who can feel neglected or overlooked by healthcare services following a dementia diagnosis. This is a disease that, at present, lacks a cure but whose burdens are manifold; there are thousands in receipt of this diagnosis that does not discriminate, and a countless army of often invisible carers. Their journey is one that we could face ourselves, and not necessarily when we are old. As we have seen within this text and the authors' previous work *The Dementia Care Workbook* (Morris and Morris 2010), carers can feel very unsupported despite the billions of pounds saved to health and social care services on account of their input. We have also seen now within this text how children can be impacted upon and experience their own unique struggles.

The authors also took the decision to base this work mainly around those experiencing young-onset dementia. Within the UK, amongst the estimated figure of 850,000 people with dementia, there are approximately 42,000 people under the age of 65 with dementia, a number that rapidly increases when taking into consideration all family members affected. A unique aspect concerning the young-onset group is the number of school age (or pre-school age) children affected. We are also looking at a group who are likely to be particularly productive in the work sphere as well as having active social and family lives. The presence of dementia within these families' lives will clearly have significant impact upon all parties involved. The focus within this work, however, is broad enough for themes and points of discussion to be extended to other personal, family or cultural dynamics and in particular those of all ages. Whilst focusing upon the family we would also ask the reader to be mindful of those with dementia who live alone and the additional burden that they might experience.

We decided that to do justice to the multiplicity of experiences of various family members we needed to address the 'journeys' embarked on individually and collectively. This involved the conceptualizing of:

- 'I am a person with dementia.'
- 'We are a couple with dementia.'
- 'We are a family with dementia.'

The experiences of family members through their dementia journey has been addressed from what we hope the reader will find a balanced (and even hopeful) perspective. This challenges the common view of progressive decline and replaces it with a picture that sees those involved moving more fluidly between positions of struggling and coping. There are now a growing number of advocates, researchers, campaigners, practitioners and resources that truly encapsulate Tom Kitwood's (1997) vision of a new and vibrant landscape for effective dementia care. We have also taken the very deliberate decision to end this work with chapters focusing upon 'Coping' and 'Dementia Champions.' It is at this point that we leave the Lawrence family to get on with their lives, encompassing Kate Swaffer's (2016) notion of *living beyond dementia*. This is not to disregard the very real distress and difficulty experienced by some families including the person with dementia perhaps needing to move into residential care or carers and family members dealing with their own complex feelings of bereavement following the person's death. We did, after much discussion, agree to end on a more hopeful note and draw the curtains across the stage whilst the family were *still* engaged in living their lives even with dementia as an ever-present entity.

We felt it appropriate to provide you with brief illustrations of our conversations as this dementia journey unfolded.

Who is the reader?

Whilst we do not know precisely who the reader might be, we wanted this work to be applicable to a broad readership. We believe that there are both personal and professional interests, sometimes intertwined with being a recipient of care services or involved in the delivery of care. As this book essentially examines family members' dementia journeys from a lived and felt experience, the information covered should be of interest and value to both families involved and health and social care personnel.

Why the Lawrence family?

The Lawrences are our fictional family serving to provide 'role prompts' for the reader in the ongoing dementia journey. The decision to 'construct' this family was taken to help to personalize themes and experiences and keep the reader more closely aligned to the lived experience. They are not designed to mirror the reader's past or present lifestyles or life choices and we deliberated long and hard as to how the family would appear and whether we would reflect aspects such as cultural mix, same-sex partnerships or other points of diversity. In the end we decided that the Lawrences would be constructed in such a way as to enable the reader to reflect against additional dynamics representing the reader's relationship or co-habitation preferences and cultural background. We have also incorporated further points concerning diversity within the text.

Why use first-person narratives?

These factual written illustrations can engender the human costs of dementia and in the latter part of this book show that dementia burdens can be challenged, and individuals, communities and national commitments can champion a cause that has its roots in stigma and prejudice. Present-day thinking provides more optimistic messages, hopeful medical and social advancements and an opportunity to relook at how we, and society, engage with the person and their dementia and their families. The reader is prompted to reflect on their thoughts and feelings when reading other people's life experiences. In essence, personal narratives promote understanding and engagement with what people are living through. They help us to better appreciate what people are expressing concerning their struggles and elements that help them to cope.

Why reflections?

Reflections have been a central tenet of this work with the reader encouraged to question, challenge or agree with the individual prompts from the range of activities and exercises provided. We have also included a series of historical observations ('How true could this be today?') from the past that informed thinking at the time, which we believe has present relevance. Our thinking around this was inspired by Tom Kitwood's (1997) *reconsidering* of the person-centred care ethos of past decades and relating it to dementia care. We believed that other past writers and researchers could also offer something for present-day care. If you are employed in dementia care services you might consider how important reflection is in your clinical practice. The structured exercises we have provided embrace a more inclusive way of learning that increases both individual and group awareness and understanding.

Essentially, this work is about better understanding the dementia experience. It is concerned with moving beyond the observed symptoms and acknowledging what a person's internal experience might entail as relating to the person with dementia, partners/carers and other family members such as dependent children. It shows that a diagnosis of dementia need absolutely not be a 'death sentence' or indeed the end of productivity. Individuals and their families need not be defined by dementia but can instead accommodate it within their continued lives, developing ways (with support and modifications) of retaining a measure of personal independence and autonomy. It acknowledges as well that within the current estimated UK figures of 850,000 with dementia, each person will have their own unique experience, something that also extends to their families.

The strong focus upon hope presented within this work may not necessarily be felt by a number of people and it is to be recognized that for some the dementia journey is indeed framed by real despair. In many cases, though, this despair and difficulty is exacerbated by the environment of care that people experience and responses they receive, which can decrease independence, feel stigmatizing and invalidating and add to the feeling of one's constricting world. This work, however, provides a reconsideration or reimagining of what the dementia journey could be for many people with their identities preserved and opportunities to have outlets for self-expression such as through artistic modes. This work also shows how powerful peer support can be, enabling individuals to feel 'heard' by those who truly understand. It also has a duality of purpose with opportunities to both receive support as well as providing this for others. There are many people and organizations worldwide acting as guides or modelling through their own lives that those affected can indeed *live beyond dementia*. We simply need to attend more fully to what we are being shown and the vibrant lessons we can learn.

References

Kitwood, T. (1997). *Dementia Reconsidered: The Person Comes First*. Buckingham: Open University Press.
Morris, G. and Morris, J. (2010). *The Dementia Care Workbook*. Buckingham: Open University Press.
Swaffer, K. (2016). *What the Hell Happened to My Brain? Living Beyond Dementia*. London: Jessica Kingsley Publishers.

Subject Index

Author Index